Beat Cancer Naturally, Now!

The Five Most Powerful Natural Alternatives to Prevent and Treat Cancer

AJAY GOEL, Ph.D., AGAF
AND TERRY LEMEROND

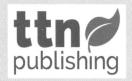

ttn
publishing

Copyright © 2023 TTN Publishing, LLC, Green Bay, WI

Library of Congress Cataloging-in-Publication Data is on file with the Library of Congress.

ISBN: 978-1-952507-32-8

Editor: Kathleen Barnes • www.takechargebooks.com
Interior design: Gary A. Rosenberg • www.thebookcouple.com

Printed in the United States of America

10   9   8   7   6   5   4   3   2   1

Contents

PART ONE

Understanding Cancer

Cancer. Even the word strikes fear in our hearts. Virtually everyone in the Western world has either had cancer or knows someone who has had this devastating disease. It is a scourge that seems to know no end. Even those lucky enough to beat cancer often fall victim to a recurrence or a spread of cancer cells months or even years later.

It seems we can't win. Even as we are gaining ground in the fight against some forms of cancer, other deadlier types of cancer are taking their place. In fact, cancer, the second greatest cause of death in the United States is rapidly gaining ground against heart disease, the Number 1 killer of Americans.

Based upon estimates by various national organizations, within the next 10–20 years, the number of cancer deaths in the United States will almost triple.

Needless to say, it's time to take this threat *very* seriously.

In this section, you'll learn what cancer is, how and why it starts and its close links to lifestyle choices and our increasingly toxic environment. In the next section, we'll explore natural ways to prevent and treat cancer.

Just a word about us:

From Dr. Goel:

I have been a cancer researcher for more than 25 years. The primary focus of my research is cancer prevention—both by developing ways to develop blood-based tests for early detection of cancers, as well as by using natural and integrative approaches to prevent, treat and improve the quality of life of patients suffering from various gastrointestinal cancers. This includes the study of colorectal, pancreatic, gastric, esophageal and liver cancers, which happen to be among some of the most common and lethal types of cancers. While I will discuss and share my research experience and understanding of these cancer types in this book, many of these results could be easily generalized to other types of cancers, which will be noted in this book when applicable.

I am currently a professor and chair of the Department of Molecular Diagnostics and Experimental Therapeutics at the Beckman Research Institute of City of Hope, Duarte, CA, associate director of Basic Sciences, City of Hope Comprehensive Cancer Center, Duarte, CA and director of Biotech Innovations, City of Hope National Medical Center, Duarte, CA. I have supervised research teams at City of Hope and other research institutions (including Baylor Scott and White Research institute, Dallas, TX) that scientifically study and validate these natural and integrative approaches to cancer. I've published more than 400 peer-reviewed scientific articles, book chapters and expert editorials on various aspects of cancer prevention including the use of natural, plant-based, integrative medicine approaches.

I can say with professional and personal enthusiasm that there is hope for people with cancer. There are new ways of approaching cancer that can prevent many types of cancer and treat established cancers.

From Terry Lemerond:

I've been in the natural products industry since 1969 when I bought a natural food store in Green Bay, WI, where I still live. It's has been a great personal pleasure for me to watch the evolution and yes, blossoming of the natural products industry and the scientific knowledge we have been able to add to ancient uses of plant medicines over those 50+ years!

I'm passionate about educating consumers and helping the natural products industry understand the vast healing benefits, indeed the treasures given to us by the plant world.

In my early years in the industry, I helped develop a wide range of standardized herbal extracts. I've contributed to the development of more than 500 natural products and learned what it takes to help people stay healthy and to regain their health if they are ill.

I've added that knowledge to also created a vast library of educational materials through my Terry Talks Nutrition website—TerryTalksNutrition.com—through newsletter, podcasts, webinars and personal speaking engagements. I've hosted a weekly *Terry Talks Nutrition* radio show for the past 30 years.

I've also written two books: *Seven Keys to Vibrant Health* (1995) and *Seven Keys to Unlimited Personal Achievement* (1997).

Please read this book carefully. We strongly urge you to copy the last chapter (For Healthcare Professionals) and share it with your doctor and others treating you or your loved ones.

CHAPTER 1

Looking at Cancer Through a New Lens

We've recently lived through a pandemic—COVID-19. It has been an emotional and physical challenge for every single one of us.

Did you realize that we've all been living through another pandemic for all of our lives and most of our parents' and grandparents' lives?

We're talking about *the cancer pandemic*. It's been with us for a very long time. Unless we become more educated about it and do something about it, this pandemic is here to stay for a long time.

President Richard Nixon declared War on Cancer in 1971. Since the early 20th century, when humans began to live longer, cancer became a scourge on our society, robbing us of the promise of lives and loved ones lost, of our productivity and of our treasure. Yes, we have made strides forward, but the cancer pandemic is still gaining ground.

The cancer pandemic is rapidly overtaking heart disease as the number one cause of death in the United States and in the Western world.

Partly because our longer lifespans give us a greater likelihood of cells going rogue, and partly because of cumulative amount of toxins taken into our bodies over our longer lives, 40% of all American men and 38.5% of all American women will have cancer sometime in their lives, says the National Cancer Institute.

Top 10 Countries with the Highest Cancer Rates*

1. Australia—452.4	6. Netherlands—349.6
2. New Zealand—422.9	7. Belgium—349.2
3. Ireland—372.8	8. Canada—348.0
4. United States—362.2	9. France—341.9
5. Denmark—351.1	10. Hungary—338.2

Top 10 Countries with the Lowest Cancer Rates*

1. Niger—78.4	6. Timor-Leste—89.7
2. Gambia—79.5	7. Tajikistan—89.7
3. Nepal—80.9	8. Djibouti—91.0
4. Bhutan—81.9	9. South Sudan—94.7
5. Congo (Rep. of)—84.4	10. Sudan—95.7

*2020 Age-Standardized Rates per 100k, WHO
Source: World Population Review, https://worldpopulationreview.com/country-rankings/cancer-rates-by-country

The latest cancer statistics say 1,668 Americans die of cancer every single day. That's 608,570 people in 2021. That's equal to the capacity of three Airbuses crashing. Every. Single. Day. Let that sink in for a moment.

They were beloved husbands, wives, sons and daughters, neighbors and friends. They are people whose lives have been squandered by a disease that we have not yet conquered. Perhaps one of them was a future president or the greatest artist since Michelangelo or The One with the key to curing cancer. The cost is heartrending.

The American Cancer Society (ACS) projected that 1.9 million Americans will be diagnosed with cancer in 2022. That does not include the common and mostly curable skin cancers, since reporting for these cancers is not required. Yet the numbers of non-skin cancer diagnoses climb inexorably higher and higher every year. The number of cancer patients who were weakened and died of COVID is unknown and will probably never be completely understood.

National costs of cancer care exceeded $208 billion in 2020. Treatment for a single case of cancer will cost an average of $150,000 according to the National Cancer Institute. Some types of cancer cost as much as $500,000 or more each year to treat. However, a majority of the patients even when treated with such expensive treatments don't respond to them and many will still succumb to their disease. If you are younger, a person of color, less educated and with a low or middle income, all the cards are stacked against you, according to the American Cancer Society.

COVID-19 was terrible and still is, but somehow the 90 million cases in the US and just over a million deaths seem pale by comparison to the cancer juggernaut that marches on, relentlessly, year by year. The Centers for Disease Control and Prevention (CDC) estimates that the number of cancer deaths will overtake those from heart disease and cancer will become the primary cause of American deaths.

What We Have Learned

We once thought that a cancer diagnosis was inevitably a death sentence, but new developments in treatment, improved screening methods and increased screening for some of the cancers help find many cancers at earlier and sometimes curable stages, changing attitudes on the part of medical professionals and a deeper acceptance of integrative therapies are credited with making many types of cancers now survivable.

This means that 16.9 million Americans with cancer are alive today because they have been cured or are in long-term remission. That means that 3.5 million Americans are alive today who would have died of cancer in 1991, as per the American Cancer Society (ACS).

The ACS says the cancer rate for adults peaked in 1991 at 215 cancer deaths per 100,000 people a year, it dropped by 32% by 2019 to about 144 per 100,000, largely because most Americans stopped smoking and because early detection and treatment has helped control the four most deadly cancers: lung, colorectal, breast and prostate.

I think that Americans are becoming more aware of cancer prevention, an important cog in the cancer containment wheel.

It's a huge advance that metastatic breast cancer is now treated as a chronic disease rather than a terminal, debilitating illness. Patients with many skin, breast and prostate cancers may live long and productive lives, an unthinkable possibility even a few years ago.

National Cancer Institute's Past Director Norman Sharpless, MD, adds that three major breakthroughs have slowed the rate of cancer deaths:

✧ **Bioindividuality:** The medical profession has now embraced the idea that each person's cancer is a unique disease and that no two cancers are alike, therefore treatments should be individually tailored. This is a huge leap forward.

✧ **Immunotherapy:** Encouraging the body's immune system and enabling it to fight cancer has now become a widely practiced fourth leg of the standard cancer treatment regimen that includes surgery, chemotherapy and radiation.

✧ **Stem cell transplants:** Intended to encourage the body to create new healthy cells to replace diseased ones, particularly cancerous cells. It's used mostly to treat leukemia, multiple myeloma and lymphoma quite successfully. The next step will likely be the routine use of stem cell transplants to prevent recurrence of cancers.

What We Haven't Learned

Dr. Sharpless has some good points, but it's not enough. The seeming light at the end of the tunnel is not enough.

While we have made some gains in the War on Cancer, and maybe even won some battles, 50 years later we are still far from winning the war.

Cancer is a terribly complex disease. The "oldthink" of treating every type of cancer identically with standardized treatments failed because cancer cells are smart. They're so smart that they almost seem to have a brain of their own. As soon as we target cancer cells from one direction, they change course and become resistant to whatever therapy worked last week or last month.

From Dr. Goel:

I've been researching cancer for nearly 30 years. I can say unequivocally that cancer is a different disease in every single case.

I've long advocated deep analysis of individual cancerous tumors. This quantum leap in our ability to analyze each person's tumor on the genetic and molecular levels also allows us to devise very specific, custom-tailored, "precision medicine" plans for each patient.

To successfully treat cancer, we must first understand the individual nature of each person's cancer. Then we must approach that cancer from a wide variety of ways. We need to *see* what will work this week and *anticipate* what will work next week. What will work in the future course of an individual's disease will assuredly be different than what has worked in the past.

Yes, there are commonalities, but cancer evolves through a complex roadmap of genes and pathways that can take on an exponential number of possibilities. Therefore, we need to approach it knowing that those smart cancer cells can adapt to the ever-evolving disease in each cancer patient with an impressive speed.

Therefore, we must pivot in our thinking and learn lessons from the modern science, which tells us that 'targeted' cancer treatments (against a single gene or pathway) that we have been using for the past two decades are only going to help the small group of patients who have early-stage cancers.

For most of our patients, we must use a multipronged approach that is broader and benefits from a 'multi-targeted' plan that can simultaneously target multiple genes and pathways, assure improved quality of life, reduce chances of cancer relapse and prolong healthy life. This is something the modern medicine currently lacks.

What's wrong with conventional cancer treatment today?

We spend exorbitant amounts of money developing new drugs that have a dismal rate of effectiveness. Some are not effective at all, yet their cost is astronomical. In order for a chemotherapy drug to receive FDA approval, pharmaceutical companies are required to prove that the drug reduces the size of tumors and can improve patient survival. However, this approach is fundamentally flawed. In the last several decades, hundreds of cancer drugs have been approved by the FDA, but more than 90% of them have not found consistent clinical use for most cancers. It is only a matter of time that these drugs are either deemed ineffective, have too much toxicity or patients

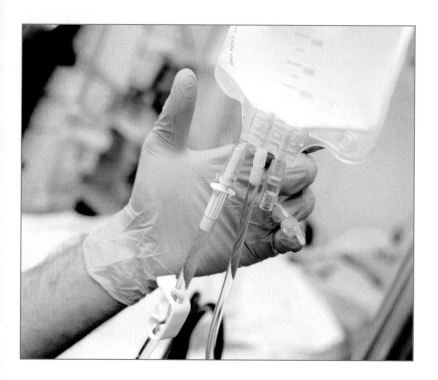

developed resistance and stop responding. In other words, such 'mono-targeted' cancer drugs have essentially failed in the grand scheme of things.

At least one study confirms that standard chemotherapy drugs are only effective in 25% of patients.

And these drugs are deadly.

Chemotherapy kills cancer patients faster than the cancer cells themselves. Let me repeat that. It is extremely important.

Chemotherapy kills cancer patients faster than the cancer cells themselves.

Here's why:

⋄ Even a tiny group of cells within a cancerous tumor can be resistant to a particular chemotherapy drug even before treatment begins.

⋄ Cancer cells can adapt and become resistant within weeks after a patient begins treatment. Sometimes resistance doesn't occur until months or even years later, but most cancers become chemoresistant.

⋄ Tumor shrinkage often does not extend a patient's life but can profoundly impair quality of life.

⋄ Individual cancers respond differently to standard drug treatments.

⋄ Chemotherapy drugs don't discriminate between cancer cells and healthy cells, so healthy cells are often damaged.

⋄ Chemotherapy targets fast-growing cancer, but not all cancer cells are fast growing.

✧ Cancer stem cells don't get killed by chemotherapy, so cancers are likely to return or spread sometime in the future.

✧ Chemotherapy damages the immune system, making it unable to disarm and remove cancerous cells from the body while potentially making it vulnerable to other infections and even other cancers.

Precision Medicine:
The Next Generation of Cancer Care

The one-size-fits-all method of delivering health care doesn't work. It never did, but until recently, we really didn't know any better.

Think of precision medicine as personalized medicine, like the old-time doctors who would bring their black leather medical bags to a patient's home and take care of whatever ailed them. Modern technology gives us the opportunity to take a deep look into a wide range of individual factors and find a specific treatment that has the best chance of working for an individual.

The Human Genome Project has unlocked a once unbelievable amount of information that helps us prevent, diagnose and treat cancer and other diseases.

Some of us have had genomic sequencing, especially those who are at high risk for certain diseases, including hormonally related cancers. Genetic analysis has made it possible for us to analyze the exact cellular components of cancerous cells from each patient and determine, project and confirm what will work for that specific disease.

In addition to genetic analysis of cancerous cells, precision medicine takes into consideration a patient's gender

PRECISION MEDICINE

Patients diagnosed with cancer	Factors contributing to the uniqueness of each person and his or her cancer	PRECISION MEDICINE

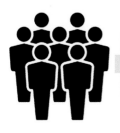

- Race / ethnicity
- Immune profile
- Metabolic profile
- Family history
- Gender and age
- Geography
- Microbiome

- Patient, tumor genome and epigenome
- Disease presentation
- Reproductive, medical factors, and comorbidities
- Lifestyle & environmental exposures
- Socioeconomic status

- Unknown factors

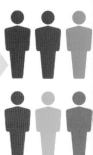

(surprisingly, something relatively new), race, age, socioeconomic status, lifestyle, family history, disease progression, metabolic profile, environment and more.

Think of it this way: If you get sick, say with the flu or high blood pressure, diabetes or cancer, conventional doctors look at a uniform treatment. They'll prescribe antivirals for flu, standard pharmaceuticals for high blood pressure, metformin for Type 2 diabetes and maybe surgery and chemotherapy for many types of cancer. This one-size-fits-all approach simply doesn't work for everybody. We have known for decades now that if you need a blood transfusion, the blood you receive must be carefully matched for a number of factors, not only to be effective, but a blood mismatch can actually be deadly.

Now we know that our genes can provide our doctors with a wealth of information about a specific and individual disease process and what will—and will not—work to treat it and cure it. The new wave of precision medicine as it applies to cancer means doing genetic tests on cancerous cells to determine what is most likely to work—and what is not—to treat that individual cancer.

In terms of prevention, precision medicine can also give a doctor an early heads up if you are at risk of certain types of cancers. We know that the vast majority of cancers are a result of lifestyle choices, so having that information in advance can head off more serious problems.

In precision medicine, gender makes a difference. Your lifestyle and diet and exercise habits make a difference. Environmental factors can even cause genetic changes based on where you grew up. Easily accessible healthcare records should also be a key part of precision medicine so doctors can look at as many individual aspects of their patients as possible.

In our reckoning, precision medicine is the future of healthcare and it should be.

WHAT YOU NEED TO KNOW . . .

❖ Effective advances in cancer treatment include immuno-therapy, stem cell therapy and the increasing willingness of conventional physicians to embrace the idea that each person is unique, and each cancer is unique in its own right.

❖ Despite some important advances in cancer treatment, cancer is likely to overtake heart disease as the Number 1 cause of death in the US by 2030.

❖ Early detection of cancers and an increased awareness of preventive measures are helping contain the cancer death rate.

❖ Every person's cancer is unique. It must be approached individually and with an ever-changing, multi-targeted treatment.

❖ Conventional cancer treatment is often ineffective and sometimes the treatment itself kills the patient.

❖ Precision medicine that looks at an individual's genetic structure and the profile of the disease itself—leads to individualized treatments and better results.

❖ Precision oncology looks at the unique genetic properties of an individual's cancer and tailors treatment based on that information.

CHAPTER 2

What Causes Cancer?

From Dr. Goel:

To put it as simply as possible, cancer results from the uncontrolled and chaotic growth of cells.

Normal body cells reproduce as perfect copies of themselves. When normal body cells start to produce inexact copies of themselves, they can be said to have mutated because DNA becomes damaged.

Remember your high school biology class? DNA is the genetic material that instructs every cell in our bodies to reproduce itself faithfully and to perform specific tasks, like forming neurons in your brain or the components of bones.

DNA instructions on cell division and other functions can be disrupted for a variety of reasons I'll go into later. When this happens, we get this wild chaotic growth that results in malignant (cancerous) tumors.

Going just a little deeper, (I promise not to overload you with too many complex scientific concepts!) we all have a few essential genes that keep cancer at bay when they are functioning properly.

Tumor suppressor genes prevent abnormal cell growth or division and *oncogenes* promote normal cell division. When either of these essential genes become unbalanced, wild cell division and cancer can occur quite rapidly.

KEY TERMS

I'm going to pause here for a moment to give you a brief glossary of terms that are important to understanding cancer:

Angiogenesis: The growth of blood vessels that feed cancerous growths.

Apoptosis: This process is also known as "programmed cell death." Each normal cell has a built-in time clock which controls the life cycle of each cell, triggers its death at a specific time point (generally a few days) and allows it to be replaced by newly formed cells. However, when old (normal) cells fail to die at the end of their lifespans and new cells continue to form, they can cluster together to form cancer.

Metastasis: The spread of cancer from one part of the body to another.

Three Primary Causes of Cancer

We're going to start this section with a bold statement: Almost all cancers are preventable and/or easily treatable if you take action early.

Many people think that cancer is hereditary. Everyone can tell you the story of colon cancer or breast cancer that "runs in families."

Yes, The Cancer Genome Atlas (TCGA) project has opened many doors, including helping us define the exact genomes that can cause cancer.

That has led to the discovery that heredity alone causes cancer in less than 2% of all cases.

If cancer or heart disease or Alzheimer's or any of these terrible diseases "run in" your family, the underlying cause is seldom what most of us would think.

These are diseases of Western civilization that are rarely the result of a hand of fate dealt by some nebulous "bad genes."

It is becoming increasingly clear that most cancers have their origins in lifestyle choices and the environment. These are the choices that "run in families," ranging from diet or alcohol and tobacco consumption, exercise habits, stress management as well as where we live, play and work every day of our lives.

We also inherit the dietary and lifestyle choices made by our parents and grandparents, but not an inherited propensity for cancer or any other disease.

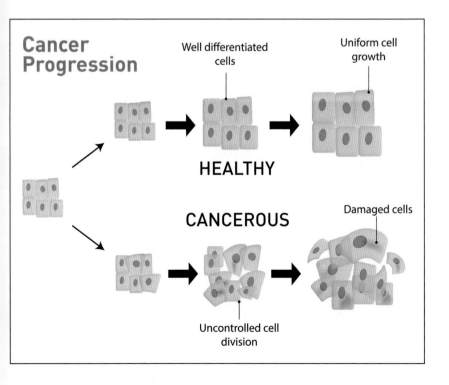

Cancer and the other chronic diseases like heart disease and Type 2 diabetes are almost entirely caused by eating too much, eating the wrong foods and living in an industrialized society that is poisoning our earth, air, water, and food.

We have control over some of these choices and for some, such as the polluted air we breathe or the tainted water from municipal systems, we do not.

Epigenetics

And yes, genes do play a role here. Our lifestyle choices can turn off cancer-preventing genes (tumor suppressor genes) and turn on cancer-promoting genes (oncogenes) in the blink of an eye (and vice-versa), a process called epigenetics. Self-destructive lifestyle choices not only affect us as individuals, but they also directly affect the gene structures of our children and their children and their children . . .

Epigenetics is a relatively new field of science. Epigenetics is a combination word meaning above and beyond genetics. Simply put, your diet and lifestyle, your caloric intake (most of us eat entirely too much!), your environment and your exposure to toxins determine how your genes work and dictate whether those genes are well-behaved or whether they go rogue. Epigenetics explains the continuously changing behavior of your gene structure, and for our purposes here, your body's genes in response to various environments.

Everything your mother did before and during her pregnancy, everything you do from the day you are born, everything you eat, drink and are exposed to in your environment has an effect on your genes.

We inherit a set of genes from each of our parents, a

combination of their genetic traits. Unless you are an identical twin, there will never be anyone else exactly like you. As you'll see in the coming pages, it's a giant lottery in which you have a great deal more control than just random luck.

As you age and grow, it is natural that some genes may get turned off—or go to sleep—as a consequence of eating habits, exercise regimens and toxic environmental stresses. Other genes that encourage uncontrolled cell growth may get turned on, thus promoting cancer growth.

When you don't eat a healthy diet or exercise regularly and you're exposed to toxins that are everywhere, including the air we must all breathe and the water we must all drink, cancer-preventing genes can go to sleep on the job, and allow diseases to take a foothold.

Unlike the small risk for hereditary cancers, cancer-related genes that are epigenetically controlled and are directly related to lifestyle choices are responsible for more than 95% of all cancers.

But here's the good news, in fact, the great news: Epigenetic changes are reversible. Unlike hereditary cancers where you have inherited a permanently defective gene, epigenetically affected genes can be easily corrected. Those changes can begin the moment you start making wiser lifestyle choices.

This is wonderful news. It highlights the promise that cancer is not our destiny. We actually have significant control on how our genes behave, as long as we are willing to make positive dietary and lifestyle choices.

Epigenetic changes are reversible.
The moment you start making wiser lifestyle choices,
you can get back on track to a healthier life.

In the next chapter, we'll be looking more deeply at epigenetics and lifestyle changes as primary ways of preventing cancer.

Other Causes of Cancer

There are a couple of other surprising causes of cancer that you might not have considered:

Obesity

A little-known and grossly underestimated cause of cancer, the obesity epidemic in the Western world is taking a heavy toll.

The soaring rate of obesity in the United States is a primary cause of death from a wide range of causes, including cancer. In 2020, 30.9% of American adults were obese or severely obese and 19% of children ages 2 to 19 were obese, 6.1% severely obese, according to the National Cancer Institute.

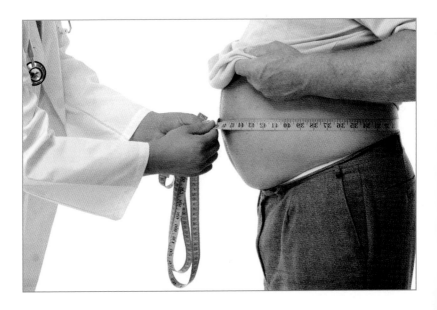

The health risks of obesity are profound: cardiovascular disease, especially heart attack and stroke, Type 2 diabetes, high blood pressure, high cholesterol, sleep apnea, fatty liver disease, asthma and chronic obstructive pulmonary disease (COPD), osteoarthritis, infertility and yes, for at least 13 types of cancer, plus an elevated risk of death from all causes.

It's estimated that about 1 in 5 cancers is directly related to being overweight.

A couple of pages back, we mentioned that most of us consume entirely too many calories. The standard nutritional recommendation for adults to consume 1,200 to 2,000 calories a day is probably way too high. Our food choices are so closely linked to huge marketing efforts by the so-called "food" industry, which entices us to eat calorically and nutritionally void concoctions that do not contribute to our nutritional needs and make us even more vulnerable to obesity and connected diseases.

Not only is obesity a direct risk factor for cancer, it also is a high risk for poor survival outcomes for those with cancer, including death. Italian researchers who reviewed studies on cancer and obesity involving 6.3 million participants found that obese people were far more likely to die of cancer, especially breast, colon and uterine cancers. It's also known that obese women are more likely to die of hormonally related cancers than normal weight women.

Let us pause here to say that many, perhaps most of us simply eat too much. It's complete nonsense to say we should eat 1,200 to 2,000 calories a day. Much of this is driven by food manufacturers who have financial interest in getting us all to eat more "food" that is high in calories and fat and devoid of nutritional value. We'll even go further and say food manufacturers want us to become addicted to "foods" that promote obesity and cancer, and heart disease and diabetes.

A diet high in fruits and vegetables that have huge nutritional value and are low in calories, add in some high-quality whole grains and perhaps a little bit of dairy, fish or meat is by far the best way to live a long and healthy life.

Losing 5% of body weight (just 13 pounds in a person who weighs 250 pounds) makes a dramatic improvement in health risks.

The National Cancer Institute says that excess body weight contributes to varying degrees of increased cancer risk depending on the type of cancer.

How obesity affects cancer risk, according to the National Cancer Institute:

◇ Fat tissue in women produces excess amounts of estrogen, a culprit in hormonally related cancers, including breast, endometrial, ovarian and some other types of cancers.

◇ High levels of insulin and insulin-like growth factor (IGF-1) found in obese people not only increase the risk of Type 2 diabetes, but they also contribute to risk of colon, kidney, prostate and endometrial cancers.

◇ The state of obesity is also a state of chronic inflammation which is a risk factor for all of the diseases mentioned above, and, for cancer, too. Inflammation causes oxidative stress, which can impair DNA and cell reproduction and create abnormal cell growth leading to cancer.

◇ Fat cells also produce hormones that can stimulate or slow cell growth and may reduce the body's ability to fight tumor growth.

✧ The lipids (blood fats) in fat cells feed cancer and can increase the aggressiveness of certain types of cancers.

Obesity significantly increases the risk of these types of cancer:

✧ Endometrial
✧ Esophageal adenocarcinoma
✧ Gastric
✧ Liver
✧ Kidney
✧ Multiple myeloma
✧ Breast
✧ Ovarian
✧ Uterine
✧ Pancreatic
✧ Colorectal
✧ *And more.*

Infections

About 13% of all cancer diagnosed worldwide are caused by infections that have not been properly treated. That's 2.2 million cases!

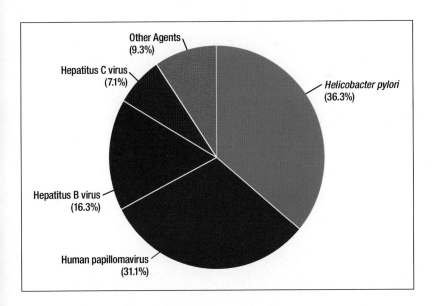

Cancer cases attributable to infections worldwide.
(2018 figures, by agent)

H. pylori

Science has shown for many years that *Helicobacter pylori*, the bacteria that causes stomach ulcers can cause stomach cancer if it is not treated.

More than one-third of cancer caused by infections are triggered by the *H. pylori* bacteria.

Treatment is fairly simple and not only cures the ulcer and the inflammation that result from the infection, it also dramatically reduces the chances that the bacteria will cause cancer, perhaps years later. Conventional medicine treats *H. pylori* infections with a two-week combination course of antibiotics and proton pump inhibitors, commonly, amoxicillin and tetracycline, and metronidazole, a simple and inexpensive therapy that will eradicate the infection as well as the risk of future cancer.

Adding specific probiotics to this regimen has been shown

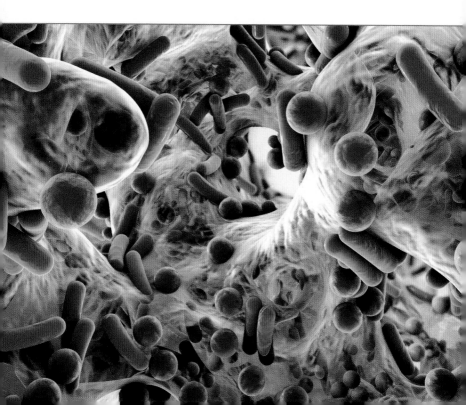

to increase the effectiveness of the pharmaceutical treatment. Treatment with lemon essential oil, ginger, and oil of oregano has been used effectively, usually along with the conventional drugs.

Some people have no symptoms of *H. pylori* infection and they have no way of knowing they have it.

Human papillomavirus

About one-third of other cancer that arises from infection are caused by the human papillomavirus (HPV), that causes genital warts. They are contagious through vaginal, anal or oral sex with someone who has the virus.

It's the most common sexually transmitted infection today and usually disappears on its own, but the virus can remain dormant in the body and, in about 10% of cases, it can emerge later as cervical cancer or other cancer of the genital region. There are several different strains of HPV, so it's important to seek a firm diagnosis if cauliflower-like genital warts appear and to be especially vigilant if it is a high-risk strain.

While there is no cure for HPV, there is an HPV vaccine that is frequently given to young men and women between the ages of 9 and 45.

HPV affects both men and women, despite the cultural narrative that it is primarily a female disease. Gay men are at particularly high risk for cancer resulting from HPV infections.

Safe sex using condoms is by far the best choice in preventing HPV.

Hepatitis B and C

These forms of hepatitis are usually transmitted through contaminated food and unprotected sex or the use of contaminated hypodermic needles, or personal items that have come into contact with the blood of an infected person like razors or nail clippers. This serious liver infection comprises about a quarter of the cancer caused by infections.

This hardy virus can survive for a month on surfaces. It can cause liver cancer. Hepatitis B is not curable, but it is preventable with vaccination.

Hepatitis C is also transmitted by contact with the blood of an infected person. Between 3 and 5 million Americans are living with the disease today. Recently, there are effective treatments and potentially cures for this virus. However, if untreated, hepatitis can cause cirrhosis of the liver, liver failure, liver cancer and even death. There is no vaccine for this strain of the virus.

There is approximately a 95% cure rate for treatment with a variety of pharmaceuticals depending on the type of viral infection you have. Treatment usually involves an 8- to 12-week course of pills that have much milder side effects than the previous injection regimen, but they are extremely expensive: $39,000 to $94,000! Insurance may or may not pay for the treatment.

UV Radiation

UV radiation or damage caused by the sun's rays, is a major cause of cancer. North America runs close behind Europe for the largest number of cancer cases caused by exposure to UV radiation. An obvious connection here is the predominance of susceptible light-skinned people in North America and Europe.

WHAT YOU NEED TO KNOW . . .

❖ Cancerous cells can be "born" when the process of programmed cell death (apoptosis) in which cells fail to reproduce exactly as their predecessor generations and have the potential to become cancerous.

❖ Genetic malfunctions that are largely driven by lifestyle choices (called epigenetics) can prevent the body's natural cancer-fighting mechanisms to turn off. Obesity, especially in women, is part of the lifestyle risk that is the underlying cause of about 20% of cancer in the US.

❖ Infections, especially untreated *Helicobacter pylori,* human papillomavirus and hepatitis B and C can lead to cancer, sometimes years later. Generally poor lifestyle choices, including dietary and exercise choices are not only the cause of heart disease and diabetes, but they are also a major cause of virtually many types of cancer.

CHAPTER 3

An Ounce of Prevention, a Pound of Cure

Cancer is a lifestyle disease in many, if not most, cases.

In the last chapter, we took a brief look at the new science of epigenetics in which lifestyle choices and toxic exposures have a profound impact on our genetic composition and can increase or decrease our risk of chronic diseases, especially cancer.

The World Health Organization says that cancer is predominantly a lifestyle disease. As far back as 2008, an iconic study from the prestigious M.D. Anderson Cancer Center declared that "cancer is a preventable disease that requires major lifestyle changes." The study says that 90–95% of cancer cases have their roots in lifestyle choices, including "smoking, diet (fried foods, red meat), alcohol, sun exposure, environmental pollutants, infections, stress, obesity and physical inactivity."

The M.D. Anderson research team estimated in 2008 that 25–30% of all cancer-related deaths were due to tobacco use, 30–35% were related to diet, 15–20% due to infections and the rest due to radiation, stress, physical inactivity and environmental pollutants.

Here's their bottom line:

"Therefore, cancer prevention requires smoking cessation, increased ingestion of fruits and vegetables, moderate use of alcohol, caloric restriction, exercise, avoidance of direct exposure to sunlight, minimal meat consumption, use of whole grains, use of vaccinations, and regular check-ups . . . Cancer is a preventable disease that requires major lifestyle changes."

We know that sounds harsh, but which is better, abandoning a couch potato lifestyle or dying of cancer? That pretty much puts it in perspective.

Epigenetics is a fundamentally fluid process. Everything about your health can change as soon as you make the right choices, allow your defective genes to reawaken and behave as they are supposed to when you were healthier.

Migration Studies

For quite some time, it was believed that people of certain ethnicities had more or less "immunity" to cancer. That turns out not to be true at all. It's a matter of lifestyle and especially of diet.

Japanese people who eat a traditional Japanese diet have among the lowest incidence of colorectal and other types of cancer in the world. However, Japanese people who immigrated to Hawaii in the 1950s and 1960s lost their near immunity to cancer within a single generation! Why? Because they adopted the unhealthy eating habits of their new country.

This is an excellent example of epigenetics and its dramatic and swift effects.

Identical Twins Validate the Science of Epigenetics

The study of identical twins is the greatest argument for the validity of the newly emerging science of epigenetics. We can all agree that identical twins are genetically identical, right? Their DNA is identical.

Yet anyone who has known identical twins knows that as they grow and age, they begin to look different. Their body types may be different. In time, they begin to develop different lifestyles and different habits. And, over time, one may develop cancer or another of the chronic diseases we've been talking about while the other does not.

Why?

This is the simplest explanation of epigenetics: diet and lifestyle choices and exposure to toxins cause some protective genes to go to sleep and may cause destructive genes to wake up or go into overdrive. When this happens, diseases can take hold. This is why one identical twin might get cancer or diabetes while the other remains healthy.

In simple terms, discovery of epigenetics helps us dispel the notion that, "Cancer is my destiny," or "Cancer cannot be prevented," simply because a family member may have had cancer. Epigenetics helps us understand that genetic or hereditary forms of most cancers are extremely rare and that most cancers can be realistically prevented or managed by making simple day-to-day changes in our diets.

Cancer is not your destiny. Cancer can be prevented by making smart dietary and lifestyle choices.

Here's another way to look at it: Genetics and epigenetics can be compared to a computer system. Genetics is the hardware and epigenetics is the software. The computer hardware (your gene structure) doesn't change, but the software (the ability of genes to behave or misbehave) can be constantly improved to enhance the performance of the computer. You can even re-write that genetic software to correct broken genetic "codes," that may be giving wrong information to your cells, causing malfunctions.

From Dr. Goel:
My Family History

My family history is an excellent example of epigenetics. I lost my father, grandfather, and grandmother to complications of diabetes. I can easily tell you that about 80% of the members of my extended family have Type 2 diabetes. Every time I return home to India for a visit, my relatives warn me to "be careful about diabetes" since it "runs in the family."

There is no question that my family is at particular risk for diabetes, not necessarily because of a genetic propensity, but because of our familial or maybe cultural eating patterns that cause those diabetes-repressing genes to malfunction.

I am proud of my Indian heritage, but our diet is extremely heavy in unhealthy white rice and fried foods. I rarely see Indian people who are extremely obese, but I see lots of lean people with big bellies. Our bone structure is meant to be lean like other Asians, but somehow some of us are able to stretch out our bellies by eating huge quantities of foods that make us vulnerable to Type 2 diabetes.

I'm very careful about what I eat and when I go back to India, I eat mostly vegetables and only a little bit of rice. On a recent trip home, I was astounded to see how many members of my family have now become obese, largely because they are adopting a more Western-style diet.

Yes, I know I am at risk for diabetes and I am doing everything I can to keep my insulin-producing mechanisms functioning properly so my genes will not go to sleep. I do not intend to become a victim of the family diabetes problem. I am careful about my eating habits.

I know for sure that I have taken every possible precaution to prevent diabetes. I have taken control. I may die of a million other things, but most likely it won't be of diabetes or its complications because I have made the choices to keep my anti-diabetes genes awake. The same is completely true for cancer.

Smoking

Clearly, smoking is still a huge issue as reflected in the death rates from cancer, which is still by far the leading cause of cancer deaths. Despite the fact that far fewer Americans smoke

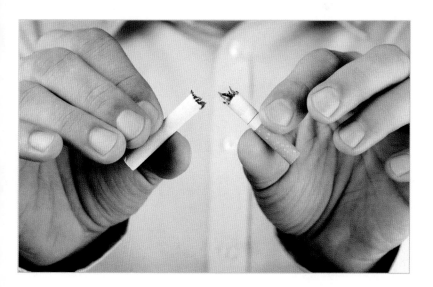

than they did 20 years ago, in 2020, approximately 12.5% of American adults still engaged in this incredibly destructive behavior, according to the Centers for Disease Control and Prevention.

Encouraging statistics from the National Lung Association note that in 1965, 68% of American adults smoked. This is a huge improvement. Nevertheless, about 32 million American adults still smoke and 16 million are afflicted with some form of lung disease. Lung cancer is the cause of 25% of cancer deaths in the U.S. Worse yet, smoking incidence among teenagers has increased.

We know. Tobacco is viciously addictive. Quitting smoking is very difficult. Some people say that kicking a tobacco habit is more difficult than quitting cocaine.

Here is our heartfelt advice: If you smoke, do whatever it takes to stop. There are behavioral strategies, patches, pharmaceuticals. Please do it today! We can guarantee this single lifestyle change will lengthen your life.

Choosing a Gene-Friendly Diet

It isn't just cultural heritage that causes genes to behave badly. Dietary patterns all over the world are the underlying causes of cancer. The Standard American Diet (SAD) is probably the most insidious choice, considering the high rates of cancer and cancer deaths in the Western world. Heavy on processed foods, factory farm-raised meats and dairy products, and light on fruits and vegetables, the SAD leaves hundreds of millions of people unnecessarily vulnerable to cancer and other chronic diseases. The SAD tells anticancer genes loud and clear that it is OK to go to sleep and wake up the cancer-producing genes.

THE ANTI-SAD DIET

❖ Eat a diet rich in fruits and vegetables, organic whenever possible.

❖ Aim for 9 servings of fruits and vegetables a day.

❖ Fill two-thirds of your plate with vegetables and whole grains.

❖ Cruciferous vegetables (broccoli, cauliflower, brussels sprouts, cabbage) contain a specific anticancer nutrient called sulforaphane.

❖ Berries, garlic, grapes, dark leafy greens all contain specific nutrients that are proven to be cancer preventive.

❖ Eat wild-caught fish at least once a week.

❖ Fatty foods are specifically risky. Minimize your meat intake, especially red meat, unless it is organic. Remember a serving of meat is the size of a deck of cards.

❖ Whole grains like brown rice, whole grain pastas and breads, and oatmeal are all important in helping manage bloods sugars and weight and managing inflammation.

❖ Keep your alcohol intake to no more than one drink a day for women and two for men.

Once you make those diet and lifestyle changes, you have the ability to turn things around, to wake up these genes, and make them do what they are supposed to do. Even in those who have already been diagnosed with cancer, such defective genes can be re-awakened and the degeneration can be minimized.

It's such an easy solution, and it's hard for us to see why more of us aren't running as fast as we can toward a healthier and leaner diet.

Other Factors

Diet isn't the only thing that may lull genes to sleep. For example, toxic exposures are definitely a serious problem.

In our increasingly toxic world, a wide variety of chemicals increase the risk of putting those crucial genes to sleep, increasing the chances of developing cancer and those other dreaded diseases.

While it is nearly impossible to avoid some of these toxins in our air and water, you can take control of some of them to minimize your exposure, including:

✧ Avoid drinking or eating from plastic cups, plates, or utensils, or storing leftovers in plastics.

✧ Minimize or eliminate your use of pesticides and herbicides in your yard and garden.

✧ Eat organic foods as much as possible to minimize pesticide exposure and GMOs in the farming process.

✧ Use natural insect repellant and sunscreens.

✧ Buy clothing that is washable; avoid dry cleaning, which is a source of toxic chemicals.

✧ If you own a home built before 1980, have it checked for asbestos.

✧ If you have a pool or hot tub, use an ozone-based filtration system or natural purification such as saltwater systems to avoid exposure to toxic chlorine or bromine.

✧ Toss out toxic household cleaners and personal care products that contain known carcinogens.

These suggestions are just the tip of the iceberg. We could write a whole book on this subject. We won't do that though, since there are numerous excellent books on natural ways to survive and thrive in a toxic world.

Exercise

Exercise is one last element of epigenetics. Don't take it lightly! There are numerous studies that prove that regular exercise keeps genes functioning as they are meant to function to prevent cancer. The more steps you take per day, the lower your risk from any cause at any age.

A pivotal study from the National Institutes of Health shows that people who walk about 8,000 steps a day reduce their risk of death from all causes, especially cancer and heart disease, by 51% over those who only take 4,000 steps a day.

We're emphasizing walking because anyone can do it and it takes minimal equipment. All you need is a decent pair of shoes. You can break up your walking regimen into just a handful of minutes at a time. Yes, walking around the supermarket and vacuuming the house count toward your daily steps!

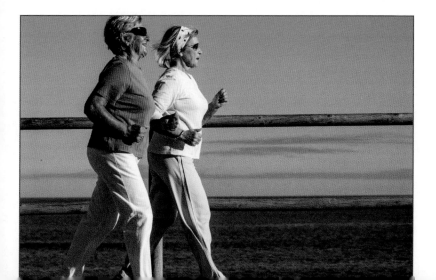

You hate walking? Try cycling, swimming, tennis, trampoline jumping. This is another of our do-whatever-it-takes recommendations for a long, healthy life.

Cancer Screening

Cancer screening has helped reduce colorectal and cervical cancer associated deaths by detecting and removing pre-cancerous lesions in the colon, rectum and uterine cervix.

Screening can also detect these and some other cancers early when treatment is often less intensive and more successful. Screening is known to reduce mortality for cancers of the breast, colon, rectum, cervix, prostate and lung cancers among people who smoke, or used to smoke.

In addition, being aware of changes in the body—such as the breasts, skin, mouth, eyes, or genitalia—and bringing them up during regular visits to your doctor, can stop an early-stage cancer from becoming a life-threatening disease.

More on Epigenetics

Epigenetics is a fundamentally fluid process. Everything about our health can change as soon as we make the right choices, allow our defective genes to reawaken and behave as they are supposed to when we were healthier.

To continue our computer analogy: We have tumor suppressive genes whose job, like the antiviral software on a computer, is to control the wild cell growth that results in cancer. We also have tumor-promoting genes that encourage out-of-control cell growth. Perfect health occurs when all these systems are perfectly balanced.

We already know that cells are programmed to be born, reproduce, and die on schedule. Anything that disrupts this life cycle can potentially cause wild cell growth and cancer.

New Cancer Drugs and Why They Cause More Problems than They Solve

The pharmaceutical industry is hard at work looking for new cancer drugs based on epigenetics. It's not doing very well for a few fundamental reasons that they don't seem to comprehend.

Here's the problem: The newer drugs take a shotgun approach and completely turn on or turn off specific genes. Now, there are some genes that are turned off when we are born, to protect us. The genes that tell tumors to grow should stay turned off. We want them to stay asleep. But these "shotgun" drugs wake up everybody, so cancer growth in one part of the body might be slowed while it might be unintentionally sped up in other parts of the body.

If these shotgun approaches completely turn off an overactive gene, this will force other genes and pathways to go haywire as they compensate for the loss of function of the gene that has been turned off by this drug. It's kind of like when you have an ancient plumbing system in your house and you replace only one of the pipes, it won't solve the problem. The new pipe may work just fine, but the old faulty system will result in leaks in other parts of the house.

Pharmaceutical drugs separate out one or two of the compounds found naturally in plants. They are built with a narrow target in mind. The drug has no way of controlling its activity, much like antibiotics that kill all bacteria in their path, taking out the good as well as the bad.

Medicinal plants have a built-in wisdom that awakens the genes that fight cancer and keeps the cancer-causing ones to stay asleep, waking up the genes that are supposed to be awake without alerting the bad guys, restoring the natural balance.

WHAT YOU NEED TO KNOW . . .

There is one huge takeaway from this chapter: Cancer is largely a lifestyle disease. It is preventable and even reversible by making wise lifestyle changes.

How to bring this about:

✜ Stop smoking!

✜ Adopt a healthy diet rich in fruits, vegetables, nuts, dried beans and whole grains, organic as much as possible, minimizing animal fats, fatty meats and processed foods.

✜ Adopt a gentle exercise program.

✜ Your genes are not your destiny!

✜ Very few types of cancer are hereditary, but lifestyle choices leading to certain types of cancer do run in families.

✜ Healthy lifestyle choices are key to cancer prevention.

CHAPTER 4

How Cancer Starts, Stays and Spreads

ancer cells are smarter than your average healthy cells. They behave in entirely unexpected ways and they will fight like fury to survive.

Anyone who has had cancer or loves someone with the disease dreads the news that the disease has spread. While it's no longer a death sentence in itself, metastasis signals the need to bring out all of the heavy artillery to fight the war on a second or even a third front.

Inflammation

It's important to recognize the deeply ingrained role of inflammation in cancer as we embark on the war against cancer in our own time. Dr. Goel's teams' recent research confirms that chronic inflammation creates a microenvironment favorable to the growth of cancer.

Cancer can be caused by any (or several) of a wide variety of things, but inflammation is definitely one of the major culprits in almost all of chronic illnesses. Inflammation triggers a cascade of events that lead to virtually every type of cancer.

Let's be sure we're on the same page here:

If you've ever whacked your thumb with a hammer or sprained your ankle, you have experienced *acute inflammation*—often characterized by redness, swelling, bruising and pain. The immune system sends out its warriors—white blood cells—to neutralize such inflammatory stress. It hurts for a while, maybe requiring a little pain medicine or ice, and then it's gone. The body heals itself and there is no lasting damage. Controlled inflammation is your body's natural response to an injury.

In contrast however, *chronic inflammation* is another thing altogether. Low-level chronic inflammation is an excessive and inappropriate inflammatory response. It is a silent killer that may have no symptoms at all. It often goes completely unnoticed.

Let's go back to some biology basics here. We promise they won't be painful.

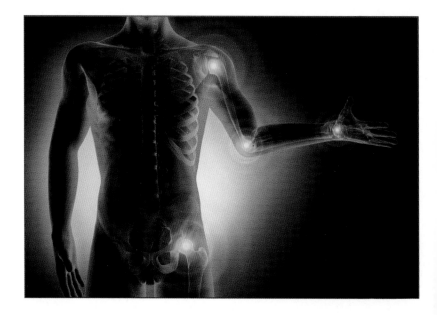

The human immune system helps defend cells and tissues from outside attacks. It fights infection and handles attacks from anything it perceives as a foreign invader. Those foreign invaders can take a wide variety of forms, including bacterial, viral or fungal infections. In general, these invaders are environmental: They are the things you put in and, on your body, the air you breathe and the water you drink.

These "invaders" (think of them as unwelcome visitors) can trigger a low level of inflammation, that can last for a long time, even decades. If it continues unchecked, it disrupts several biological functions, including the all-important immune system.

NF-Kappa B is a cellular process that controls inflammation inside cells. It is the hub of inflammation. Without going into deep scientific explanation, it's important to know that NF-Kappa B is an inflammation-causing protein that is intimately linked to the way hundreds of other genes eventually behave. In most healthy cells, NF-Kappa B levels are very tightly controlled. But sometimes, it becomes overactive and upsets the inflammatory balance, almost like an allergic reaction. Eventually, the long-term inflammation triggered by NF-Kappa B hyperactivity can cause and promote cancer.

Chronic inflammation can also be caused by the same lifestyle choices we've talked about:

✦ Eating processed and adulterated foods

✦ Overeating

✦ Smoking

✦ Breathing polluted air

✦ Drinking municipal water

◇ Using toxic personal care products (shampoo, soap, tooth-paste, makeup, deodorant and more)

◇ Toxic cleaning products

◇ Petrochemicals and gas fumes

◇ Pesticides and herbicides

◇ Living and working in toxic environments (among them off-gassing carpets, furniture and bedding)

If you are obese, or have diabetes, heart disease, Alzheimer's, osteoporosis, depression or cancer, you have a disease triggered by chronic inflammation. If you don't have any of these diseases yet, count yourself lucky, be proactive about it and do what you can to prevent or minimize your levels of inflammation.

The Role of Chronic Stress in Inflammation

Long-term unrelieved stress is another important cause of chronic inflammation. Who doesn't experience stress on a daily, perhaps even hourly basis these days? Sometimes we don't even recognize it, but we are actually stressed by the small day-to-day stuff like getting kids to school, meetings, a work deadline or getting stuck in traffic, not to speak of major ones like pandemics that completely upend our lives. Each of these stressors can trigger chronic inflammation.

The human body is designed to respond to threats with a cascade of biological events that give us superhuman strength. Imagine this: Your toddler has wandered into the street. You feel that surge of adrenaline. You run faster than you ever

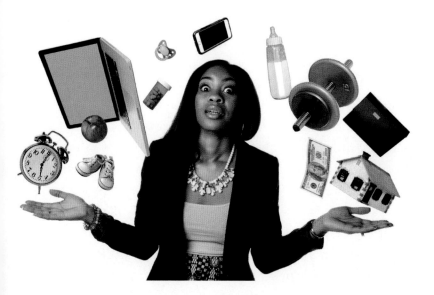

imagined possible. You dart between cars, heart pounding, your brain laser focused and hyper alert. When you finally grab onto the precious little one, you exhale a huge sigh of relief, unaware that you had been holding your breath. When you finally bring her to safety, you sink to the ground, relieved and exhausted.

Without being aware of it, you've just demonstrated the instinctive stress and release response ingrained in the human race since the beginning of our species.

Biologically, when there is an acute stress situation, your adrenal glands release a flood of adrenaline, cortisol and other chemicals that shut down every bodily system that is not needed for survival in the next few minutes. Digestion is slowed. Wound healing is put on hold. Your liver releases stored glucose for energy.

So just like acute inflammation that we discussed a few pages back, saving your child from traffic is a threat that has a beginning, middle and an end. It takes place in a few seconds, a minute at most.

Our ancestors dealt with frequent life-threatening situations. Most of these crises ended with a time of rest, recovery, relaxation and relief.

Now let's switch gears to today's world. We rarely experience life-threatening threats, yet stress just keeps piling on us, unrelieved, hour after hour, day after day. While you might not often feel the heart-pounding superhuman powers of the threat of your child wandering in traffic, your body is responding in exactly the same way, even if the threat is only your child's poor grade on a test, a looming deadline at work, or an argument with your spouse.

And—here's the important part—we don't take the recovery time our bodies and minds desperately need. Voila! Chronic stress. And chronic stress is the mother of chronic inflammation.

What happens when you have chronic inflammation?

We've already mentioned that chronic inflammation compromises the healthy immune system, among the many destructive effects it has on the human body.

It also causes the production of free radical oxygen molecules, which damage the DNA of cells. The DNA is a blueprint on how to make a new cell. If the blueprint is damaged, the new cell is defective. It may even be mutated into a cancer cell.

These inflammatory triggers—perceived as foreign invaders by your immune system—start a slow cascade that opens you to a variety of diseases.

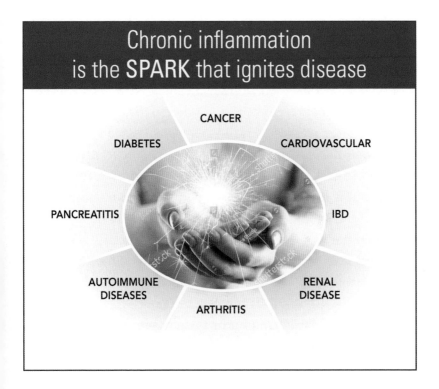

Chronic inflammation is the **SPARK** that ignites disease

A strong, healthy immune system can easily handle an invader, whether it's the flu virus or even the occasional Big Mac attack. But over a lifetime, the foreign invaders begin to pile on, weakening your immune system.

Then these invaders begin to search for weak points and gradually they find a way to cause mutations in critical genes. Your weakened immune system is a defense mechanism with no way to repair the damage to one or two or several thousand genes, or even to millions of cells, so they continue to multiply. The seed is sown.

Many things begin to go awry.

Every cell has a definite lifespan, and this process is very efficiently regulated by *apoptosis* or programmed cell death (we'll take a deeper dive into that in a couple of pages. A compromised immune system can affect the genes that control such death signals. Cells that don't get those death signals live on and on, far beyond their normal lifespan. New cells continue to be born, while the old cells don't die, so the cells continue to pile up in large masses. This old-cell logjam essentially leads to formation of tumors and cancers.

The old-cell logjam doesn't always lead to formation of cancer, but it can have other effects in other parts of the body as well. For example, if old cells become rooted in the pancreas, they can interrupt the natural renewal of islet cells, eventually damaging the body's ability to produce insulin and causing Type 2 diabetes. In the brain, the inflammation can impair the function of neurons and result in Alzheimer's disease.

We said at the beginning of this chapter that cancer cells are incredibly smart. We are well aware that it is not scientifically sound, but it's almost like these evil little creatures have brains. They thwart virtually every type of treatment we try. They shuffle nutrients away from other parts of the body and divert blood supplies for their own growth. They even grow new blood vessels to feed themselves and ensure their survival, a process called *angiogenesis*.

Deadly Drugs to Combat Chronic Inflammation

Can't we just take some sort of drug to combat chronic inflammation?

We wish the answer was that easy, but sadly, it's not.

You've no doubt heard of NSAIDs—non-steroidal anti-inflammatory drugs. That's just scientific jargon for drugs used to treat inflammation, fever, and pain. This includes over-the-counter medicines like aspirin, ibuprofen and naproxen (Aleve) and diclofenac (Voltaren) topical gel as well as prescription medicines like celecoxib (Celebrex), piroxicam (Feldene), diclofenac (Cambia, Cataflam, Voltaren and more), oxaprozin (Daypro) and several others.

These drugs, prescription or not, belong to a class called cyclooxygenase or COX 1 and 2-enzyme pathway inhibitors, which are intended to block inflammation. We won't drag you through a complicated scientific explanation for all of that except to say that these are systems that should not be disrupted or blocked.

It might seem like blocking inflammation would be a good thing, but some anti-inflammatories extract a high cost.

There are several serious health consequences for people taking NSAID drugs, some of them even caused by short-term use:

✧ Doubled risk of heart attack and stroke

✧ Doubled risk of death from heart attack or stroke

✧ Triple the risk of gastrointestinal bleeding, sometimes fatal

✧ Gastric ulcers

✧ Kidney failure

✧ Liver failure

✧ Blood thinning leading to prolonged bleeding after surgery or injury

In fact, as many as 16,500 deaths each year and more than 100,000 hospitalizations are attributed to the gastrointestinal complications of long-term use of NSAIDs in the U.S. alone.

It is simply not safe to take these drugs every day to relieve chronic inflammation, even though doctors commonly prescribe these drugs, and you can find them on any drugstore shelf.

Please avoid them and talk to your doctor about your desire to avoid their use whenever possible.

Now let's go into each of these major fronts where we can address cancer individually and see how we can use various natural remedies to prevent and even reverse these key elements of cancer.

Apoptosis: Cells that Refuse to Die

The formal explanation for apoptosis is programmed cell death. You have 70 trillion cells in your body, give or take a few. Each one has a specific life span. Each cell is born, an exact replica of its parent cell. It matures, reproduces creating offspring that are exact replicas of itself, and, if it is working correctly, eventually it dies.

When the cell dies, the body releases specific proteins that break down the cell walls and the RNA (ribonucleic acid—genetic material) from the old cell, which shrinks and sends out a signal to the body's vacuum cleaners called macrophages to seamlessly dispose of it, leaving no trace.

However, sometimes things go wrong. The instruction manual inside the cell gets damaged, and the instructions for apoptosis are blotted out. There are too many living cells. The old cells that refuse to die become nearly immortal. In addition, old cells may have impaired genetic programming, so when they do reproduce, they may not make identical copies of themselves as nature intended. Old cells and newly formed young cells that are reproducing wildly pile up. Instead of

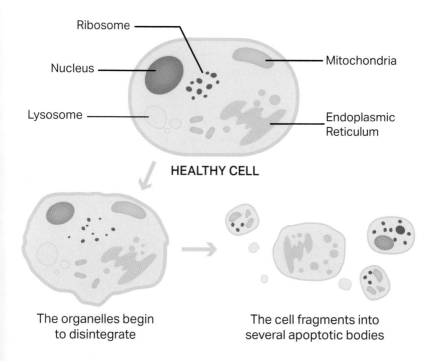

Ribosome

Nucleus

Lysosome

Mitochondria

Endoplasmic Reticulum

HEALTHY CELL

The organelles begin to disintegrate

The cell fragments into several apoptotic bodies

being flushed out of the system as happens naturally when cells die, these impaired and hyperactive cells form tumors, individually or in partnership with each other.

Remember, we said that cancer cells are smart. They have figured out a way to make themselves immortal and to resist the body's chemical death signals. They also can themselves trigger complicated genetic changes to escape apoptosis.

Some of these cancer cells are even resistant to conventional medicine's efforts to kill them. There are drugs that are geared toward causing those nearly immortal cells to die, but like most pharmaceuticals in the cancer industry, these drugs not only kill the cancer cells, but kill the normal cells as well, which is one of the reasons for the toxicity and side effects patients experience when they undergo chemotherapy.

Angiogenesis: Fierce Survivalists

The term comes from the two Greek words *angio*, meaning blood vessels and *genesis* meaning beginning. In a positive sense, angiogenesis is a crucial part of the development of a baby in the womb as it grows, creating a circulatory system to support critical organs like bones, skin and brain. Angiogenesis continues throughout our lives, usually for good purposes, like healing wounds or repairing damage.

It's part of a delicate balance between normal and healthy blood vessel growth intended to keep the body nourished and the destructive network of tiny blood vessels called capillaries that feed malignant tumors.

Those tumors begin with abnormal clumping of cells that didn't get the messages that it was time to die. Now they have become expert survivalists.

In their urgent quest to survive, the tumor cells release a specific set of chemical signals that command the body to produce a network of blood vessels that will feed the tumor, provide it with nutrients and oxygen, ensuring its ability to survive, grow and thrive. These selfish cancer cells then are able to shuttle nutrition and oxygen from healthy cells to feed themselves.

Once a tumor has established its own blood vessel network, it becomes immeasurably stronger. It can easily send signals to develop further development of enhanced circulation to feed even more and larger tumors. Treatment becomes far more difficult.

What we want to do is to induce tumor "hypoxia"—to literally starve the tumor by cutting off its oxygen and nutrient supply.

Some types of cancer therapy target these abnormal blood

vessels, working on the theory that cancerous tumors cannot grow beyond about the size of a pinhead without a blood supply.

Recently developed therapies include a relatively new class of drugs called angiogenesis inhibitors that are intended to starve tumors to death. They work—for a small percentage of patients—by blocking the signals sent by those brilliant cancer cells calling for blood supply.

The handful of drugs designated for this purpose have serious side effects, as do most chemotherapy drugs, including high blood pressure, risk of stroke or heart attack, gastrointestinal perforations (a rupture of the stomach or intestine), slow wound healing, severe bleeding and birth defects.

Metastasis: Alien Invaders

Metastasis is the spread of cancer from a primary site to another. It's the third leg of the stool that explains how cancer starts, gets a foothold and kills.

Here's what happens and how metastasis is connected to apoptosis and angiogenesis:

Those immortal cells (the result of a deficiency of the natural process of apoptosis) have clumped together to form tumors. Then they have developed their own food delivery mechanism (angiogenesis) and finally, they find a way to spread themselves throughout the body (metastasis) to ensure their survival.

There is a second stage of angiogenesis, called lymph angiogenesis, in which the blood vessels surrounding the tumor begin to migrate into the lymphatic system. (You may recall from your high school biology that the lymph system is a vast network of vessels and a vital part of the immune system that constantly sweeps bacteria and other pathogens out of the body.)

The cancer cells are able to travel through the lymphatic system, eventually winding up in lymph nodes. From there it's an easy trip from the lymphatic system to the bloodstream, and then they can go wherever they want. That explains how cancer can spread to distant organs, for example from the ovaries to the lung or from the breast to the bones or brain.

In short, angiogenesis insures the survival of the cancer cells in the short-term. Metastasis promotes long-term survival of the cancer and gives it the opportunity to invade many organs.

Of course, these metastases are what will eventually kill the human body. In the process, the death of the body will also mean the death of the tumors, but the metastasizing cells aren't all that smart in the end or that predictive to recognize that their strategy winds up being fatal for both the host and the cancer.

Metastasis: How Cancer Spreads

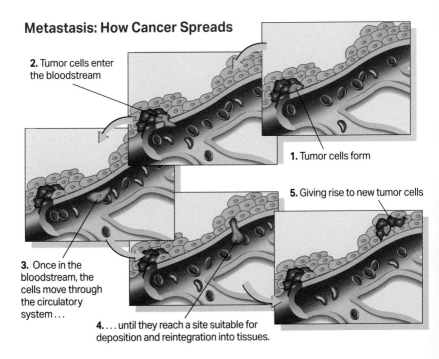

2. Tumor cells enter the bloodstream

1. Tumor cells form

5. Giving rise to new tumor cells

3. Once in the bloodstream, the cells move through the circulatory system...

4.... until they reach a site suitable for deposition and reintegration into tissues.

WHAT YOU NEED TO KNOW . . .

So, we have a spiral here—or a vicious circle if you like:

Chronic inflammation begins the cycle of cellular mutation that results in chronic disease, including cancer.

Apoptosis allows cells to live beyond their natural lifespan.

Angiogenesis creates life-giving nutrient networks to feed those bundles of cancer cells and allows them to grow.

Metastasis, creating new tumors in other parts of the body, which build up more masses of cancer cells, and new nutrient networks, and new metastases that will eventually kill the host human if the cycle is not broken.

CHAPTER 5

Stop Cancer from Returning

By reading this far, you've probably come to some of the same conclusions we have.

First is that we must all recognize that cancer cells are the geniuses of the biochemical world. They're undoubtedly smarter than your average brain, bone or skin cell. Cancer cells are driven for self-preservation, with strength far beyond the survival instincts of normal cells. Like all life forms, they fight like demons to survive, but they are also incredibly intelligent, enough to thwart most attempts to kill them. It's almost like they have their own brains.

You'll note I said, "most," but not "all" attempts to kill them.

Here are three new areas for us to examine:

✧ **Cancer stem cells**: Super cells that govern other cancer cells and are astonishingly difficult to kill.

✧ **Chemoresistance**: Cancers that become resistant to chemotherapeutic drugs that were effective earlier in the disease process.

✧ **Chemosensitization**: Making cancer cells more receptive to accepting the drugs that will eventually kill them.

Cancer Stem Cells

We've already established that most of us know someone who has had cancer. You probably already know that even with the standard cancer treatments—surgery, chemotherapy and radiation, or any combination of these—cancer often returns. It may be three or four years or even longer, but those resistant cancer cells find a way to hide and survive, and some eventually emerge again and thrive. These are *cancer stem cells* and they can be deadly. When cancers return, they tend to be far more vicious and more aggressive than they were the first time around.

When a child is conceived, the egg and the sperm divide into a handful of healthy stem cells. Stem cells are the point of origination for all tissues in the body. Malleable like a child's Play-Doh, stem cells can become any kind of cells. They can be brain cells, heart cells, pancreas cells, skin cells or hair and nail cells. Stem cells are the superheroes of the body, capable of unlimited potential.

Cancer stem cells are different. We are not born with cancer

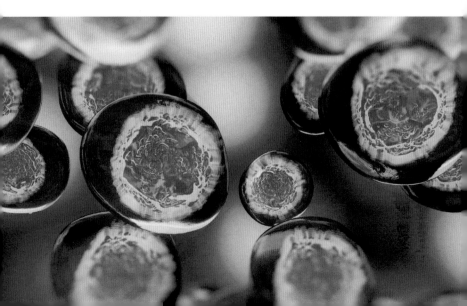

stem cells. They are a tiny subset of cancer cells themselves. They are called this because they can be the point of origination for a cancer recurrence or disease relapse. They can disguise themselves and lie low, avoiding chemo and radiation therapy. Then when the coast is clear, they can spring forward and start making cancer cells again.

Cancer stem cells initiate and maintain cancer and contribute to recurrence and chemotherapy drug resistance. Almost like the multi-tasking white-hatted miRNAs that combat cancer, these are their alter-egos, super-cells that govern other cancer cells and command them to grow and proliferate.

Cancer stem cells are immortal—or nearly so. Think of them as super-cells. As we've learned in earlier chapters, cancer cells do not have a normal lifespan like healthy cells. They live on and on, reproducing in their twisted fashion, creating more cancer cells and larger tumors that spread throughout the body.

In addition, these cancer stem cells have an uncanny ability to hide from conventional medicine's diagnostic "radar," hiding in the deepest recesses of the body, appearing to sleep or staying quiet for months, even years, before they awaken and begin to grow again with a vengeance.

The scientific community is in general agreement that targeting cancer stem cells is "a very promising concept and therapeutic option to eradicate tumors and prohibit resistance and recurrence." However, this is a tall order to achieve. Until now, we don't have any modern cancer drugs that can successfully target cancer stem cells. This is why we see so many cancer patients who think they are cured and then later experience cancer recurrence, sometimes at the same site and sometimes in another part of the body.

Chemoresistance

In all Dr. Goel's years of cancer research, he has seen almost every cancer patient develop some degree of resistance to chemotherapy drugs.

This means that chemotherapy drugs that were effective in the earlier phases of treatment almost always stop working over time. The tumors become resistant to the drug's intended effects and cancer cells continue to grow unchecked.

These cancer cells can be fooled once if they've never been exposed to a chemo drug before. The drug may destroy 95% or more of the cancer cells. The cells the chemo does not kill are the ones left to reproduce. The cancer becomes resistant to that drug. Regardless of what we throw at them, they figure out a way to develop resistance to one drug after another until we have nothing else to offer.

You already know that cancer cells have a hyper-survival mechanism. In simple terms, they don't want to die. Remember our examination of apoptosis, or programmed cell death? Well, many chemo drugs target the apoptosis pathways, reminding those nearly immortal cancer cells when it's their time to die.

Over time, those genius cancer cells figure out a way to shut down the message. They overrule the command to bring back the natural pattern of cell death, allowing the cancer to continue to grow and spread.

Of course, they also are able to overcome the command to stop supplying nutrients to the cell clusters and blood vessel nutrient networks, overcoming all efforts to starve them.

Didn't we tell you these cancer cells were smart?

Cancer stem cells are even stronger and more resistant to conventional therapies than those foot soldier cancer cells.

So, the patient has already undergone at least one course of chemotherapy, complete with myriad side effects that can include nausea, hair loss, weight loss, muscle wasting, extreme fatigue, organ damage and more, only to learn that the cancer has returned.

The only option most doctors can offer is another course of chemotherapy with a different drug, administered in the hope that the new drug will trick the genius cancer cells into committing suicide.

The vicious circle has been set. Some of the cancer cells will die, but, until now, there have always been survivalist cancer cells that will hide out in the physiological wilderness and come back again another day.

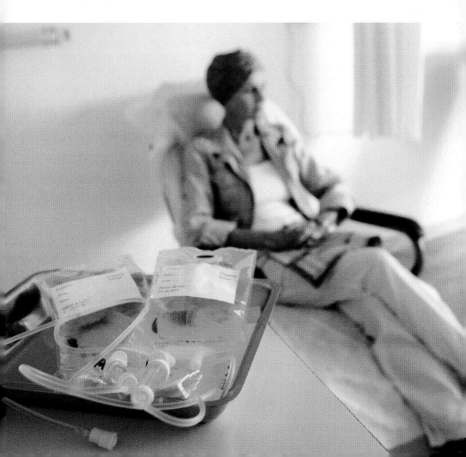

Cancer very often returns, perhaps in the same place, perhaps in another part of the body. Doctors try another form of chemo. The patient weakens. Quality of life deteriorates to the point where it becomes intolerable. The outcome has been set almost from the beginning: The doctors eventually announce they can offer nothing else to overcome those cancer cells. The patient, in utter despair at the thought of more life-consuming drugs, loses hope.

It's a horrible story that too many of us have witnessed, if not experienced for ourselves. It's heartbreaking and it doesn't have to be this way at all.

What causes chemoresistance? You've probably already got a good idea: Those cancer stem cells with their superpowers are able to escape, evolve and hide from all known chemotherapy drugs.

Chemosensitization

This is a glass half full/glass half empty topic. Chemosensitivity or chemoenhancement is the opposite of chemoresistance. It means that some botanicals actually help sensitize cancer cells, specifically those notoriously tough cancer stem cells, making them vulnerable to destruction by chemotherapy drugs, ending their resistance, and allowing them to be killed by the drugs.

Chemosensitivity also means that cancerous cells can be targeted by chemotherapy drugs while healthy cells remain unharmed. This is an important factor in cancer treatment, since when healthy cells are damaged, so is the immune system, leaving a cancer patient with increased vulnerability to all sorts of infections, including those we know cause cancer.

WHAT YOU NEED TO KNOW . . .

❖ **Stem cells:** We're adding a new component to the vicious circle of cancer. These cells have a super-enhanced will to live and are able to overcome almost all efforts to kill them known to conventional medicine. Their ability to escape detection is the primary reason why most cancers recur after conventional treatment.

❖ **Chemoresistance:** Cancer cells, and particularly cancer stem cells, are able to become resistant to chemotherapy drugs in only a few generations, so chemotherapy no longer works after a period of time. Eventually, doctors run out of options.

❖ **Chemo-enhancement:** Some botanicals have their own superpowers, not only to overcome chemoresistance, but to actually make conventional chemotherapy drugs work better with less damage to healthy cells.

Stay with me. You'll learn all about these botanicals with superpowers in the coming pages.

PART TWO

Botanicals that Combat Cancer

Introduction

We hope the first section has given you some insight into the challenges of preventing and treating cancer. Ideally, of course, you never get cancer in the first place because you've adopted a life-affirming healthy diet and lifestyle that makes cancer a remote possibility.

But, for whatever reason, you or someone you love has been diagnosed with cancer. What's next?

In this section, we'll take a close look at five natural ways to address cancer, each with its own specific and powerful properties. Some of them, when combined, have a synergistic effect, meaning that each enhances the other in new and better ways. In simple terms, 1 + 1 = 3 or even 1 + 1 = 5. Does that seem confusing? It's new math.

Let us give you a brief explanation of botanicals and why they are unique treatments for a variety of diseases.

Plants are comprised of a complex array of dozens, sometimes even hundreds, of different compounds. Each is unique. Each works in its own way, synchronizing with other components of the same healing plant.

Well-meaning scientists, seeing that one fraction of the plant, might be effective for a certain purpose in a laboratory, erroneously try to formulate a drug based on that single element. For example, we know that curcuminoids in curcumin have anticancer effects, it doesn't stand to reason that these substances could be extracted from the plant with the same effects. More about that coming up in the next chapter.

What they are missing is the support the dozens of other elements of the plant molecule contribute to the total healing power. Separating out one element is like chopping off three legs of your chair and expecting the single remaining leg to support you. It just doesn't work.

There's another element that is important in this picture: Plant compounds cannot be patented. This means that drug companies need to create something artificial and new so they can make profits. This should be all we need to say to help you understand the machinations pharmaceutical companies use to create those staggeringly expensive chemotherapy drugs (and other prescription drugs) that have questionable benefits.

In the coming chapters, we'll be looking at three complex healing plants with which Dr. Goel has done extensive research, what each one contributes to cancer prevention, treatment and reversal, and how powerfully they can work in combination.

We'll also take a deep dive into melatonin, which is not a plant, but a quasi-hormone that is absorbed through the digestive system from a wide variety of foods, including many fruits, vegetables, grains, nuts, seeds, eggs and fish. Since, by definition, no hormone is absorbed through food, melatonin cannot be accurately described as a hormone or specifically plant based. It's a compound that we know has powerful anti-cancer properties.

CHAPTER 6

Curcumin

We're putting curcumin right at the top of this section because it is the powerhouse, the macdaddy of botanicals that prevent, address and even reverse cancer. I can say this with great confidence because I have spent decades of my professional career researching and confirming the healing effects of curcumin for a variety of diseases, but mostly cancer.

The results have been enormously exciting because science now confirms that curcumin is an effective preventive and treatment for *every* single disease for which it has been studied.

Its anti-inflammatory, antioxidant, antimicrobial and anti-cancer properties are unique in the plant world. That's what makes curcumin the ideal botanical medicine to conquer virtually every type of cancer and many chronic diseases.

What Is Curcumin?

So, what is curcumin? If you love curry, you're no doubt familiar with turmeric, the vivid orange-colored spice that gives curry its distinctive flavor. Inside the turmeric rhizome (root) is a compound called curcumin, perhaps the most powerful botanical-derived, natural medicine known to humankind.

However, as healthy as turmeric is as a spice, it has a very low curcumin content. Unless you were born into a culture that

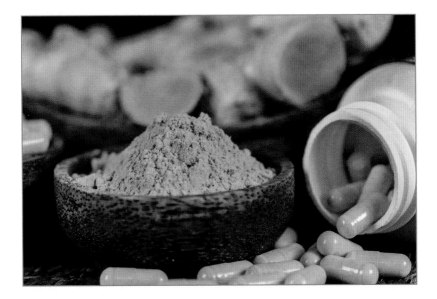

consumes turmeric-laden meals three times a day as part of your daily diet for your entire life, you're unlikely to get any real health or medicinal benefit from consuming an occasional meal containing this tasty spice. (BTW, curcumin and cumin are very different botanicals. It's easy to confuse them. It's curcumin you want.)

The curcumin content of turmeric is only 2 to 5%, depending upon the species of turmeric, and the climate and soil where it is grown in different parts of the world. Although turmeric may be the most natural way of achieving health benefits of curcumin, such an approach is not practical for those who can't consume enough turmeric on a daily basis for a lifetime. That's why turmeric is not likely to be anywhere close to as effective as curcumin for prevention or treatment for cancer or the other diseases we're talking about. Curcumin is many times more powerful than turmeric.

Turmeric is the spice and curcumin is the medicine.

Turmeric is the healthy food. Curcumin is the medicine.

This humble herb, used in India for millennia, has no known serious side effects and no toxicity level, even when taken in reasonably large amounts.

Turmeric has been an integral part of the religious traditions and customs of India's predominantly Hindu culture for more than 6,000 years. Dr. Goel's compatriots in India eat large amounts of turmeric several times every day in their favorite curry dishes.

Cancer rates in India are very low, probably due to the universal consumption of turmeric and other medicinal herbs and spices people eat as part of their daily diet several times a day for a lifetime. About 1.4 million cases of cancer were reported in India in 2020 in a population of 1.3 billion. That means cancer is rare in India, affecting about 94 cases per 100,000 people. Compare that to the shockingly high U.S. cancer rate of 439 every 100,000 people, a rate 4.5 times higher than in India.

They're certainly doing something right in India, although it's interesting to note that the cancer rate is projected to increase in the coming years, in part due to the increasing popularity of Westernized diets. Dr. Goel has no doubt that traditional Indian diet has provided protection against cancer and other dreaded diseases. If his compatriots would continue to eat a traditional diet, he has no doubt their cancer protection would remain in place.

Why Conventional Cancer Drugs Don't Work

Allow us to take a quick side trip here to elaborate on the shortcomings of conventional medicine, which continues to focus on single-pathway medicines, especially cancer medicines.

Many scientists have gone to great lengths to isolate active molecules (or medicines) from natural plant-based compounds. Nearly 75% of all approved anticancer drugs are derived from natural plant-based compounds or mimic certain aspects of the plant one way or another. As an aside, approximately 25% of all prescription drugs used in the U.S. are derived from plants.

However, these drugs, even the ones based on plants, are developed to address single-target pathways.

Mother Nature is brilliant. Complex natural plant-based compounds, like curcumin, have the ability to target not just one gene or pathway, but to simultaneously control many different pathways. Such multi-targeted therapies, attack cancer cells from many directions all at once and reduce their ability to survive and thrive.

Curcumin's multi-pathway power has been validated in thousands of scientific studies. Though other botanical medicines have been tested and a few have some multi-targeting properties, none compares to the strength of curcumin and its ability to address so many cancer genetic pathways at one time. This wide-ranging approach is far more effective in combatting this complex disease than the mono-targeted, modern, designer, chemotherapeutic drugs conventional medicine has unsuccessfully used for the past several decades.

Curcumin's Broad-Based Attack Against Cancer

Curcumin addresses multiple mechanisms for cancer cell creation, communication with healthy cells and the survival of cancer cells. I've talked about epigenetics, apoptosis, angiogenesis, and metastasis in previous chapters. Curcumin addresses all of these and more.

One of the many elements of curcumin's power was verified in my 2022 study that showed curcumin helps rebalance the gut microbiome (the trillions of healthy and unhealthy bacterial, fungal and viral components in the human gastrointestinal system). This not only promotes general health benefits, but specifically re-establishes microbial balance that can be lost for a variety of reasons. It prevents leaky gut syndrome, a means by which gut bacteria can travel to other parts of the body and cause disease.

Among the pivotal studies that confirm curcumin's value as a cancer preventive and treatment is my team's 2009 finding that curcumin actually enhances the effectiveness of a variety of chemotherapy drugs used to treat a wide variety of the deadliest cancers.

Plus, it increases the effectiveness of radiation therapy treatment.

Newer research confirms that curcumin convinces cancer cells to destroy old, damaged and defective cell parts and prevent them from becoming cancerous, a process called autophagy.

Not only that, we also were able to prove that curcumin overcomes the tendency of "smart" cancer cells to resist conventional cancer treatments and protect healthy cells from the dire side effects of chemotherapy, so that smaller amounts of the drugs are needed.

Best of all, curcumin is one of the few, rare medicines, natural or otherwise, proven to eliminate cancer stem cells that are resistant to chemotherapy drugs. They can remain dormant, even when a patient recovers and is declared "in remission," only to have a recurrence of cancer in the same place or elsewhere, perhaps years later.

Curcumin steps in to interrupt the best-laid plans of genius cancer cells.

It has been scientifically proven to convince those unique master cells—cancer stem cells—to die at the right time.

This is a huge and exciting step forward in cancer treatment, buried in the usually dry and unemotional scientific jargon from the National Cancer Institute. Curcumin may well be the most powerful substance known to science when it comes to eradicating cancer stem cells.

Will curcumin eliminate the cancer stem cells forever? Maybe yes, maybe no. We have studied this aspect of curcumin for several years and, while we need more research, Dr. Goel feels quite optimistic that ongoing and future studies of curcumin in humans will show us that curcumin can provide a cure or a much, much longer remission time than we now know.

Curcumin: The Anti-Inflammatory Powerhouse

We've mentioned the destructive effects of chronic inflammation. We'll add here that curcumin is the most potent anti-inflammatory botanical substance known to science.

Curcumin works as an anti-inflammatory to prevent the growth of cancerous cells in a variety of ways.

1. It inhibits the COX-2 and NF-Kappa B inflammatory pathways, preventing chronic inflammation.

2. It scrubs away the free radical oxygen molecules that promote the growth of arachidonic acid, a hormone that has been called "the mother of inflammation."

3. It controls the body's production of cytokines, proteins that serve as molecular messengers between cells. When there are

too many pro-inflammatory cytokines, chronic inflammation is the ultimate consequence.

4. It slows or stops the production of certain enzymes, such as protein kinase, that increase inflammation.

Chronic inflammation is the spark that ignites the disease.

If all of this science is a bit confusing, not to worry. **It's just important to know that curcumin works in four distinctly different, but powerful ways, to stop chronic inflammation that has been linked to cancer and other diseases commonly associated with the aging process.** This means that cancer can't get a foothold. Without chronic inflammation, there is no distorted reproduction of damaged cells that can eventually turn into cancer cells.

Antioxidant Punch

Curcumin is also by far the most powerful antioxidant known to science, hundreds of times more powerful than blueberries and dark chocolate, which have substantial antioxidant capabilities themselves.

Curcumin literally scrubs the oxidative "rust" from cells, preventing serious disease and reversing diseases you may already have. It helps stop cell deterioration and restores the cellular genetic codes to more youthful levels, ensuring those cells will reproduce more like they did when you were young, which helps to prevent cancer and many other diseases associated with aging.

On the ORAC (Oxygen Radical Absorbance Capacity) scale that rates the antioxidant power of foods, curcumin has been rated over 15,000 in one single gram, while antioxidant-rich blueberries have only a 600 ORAC rating per gram.

Of course, this doesn't mean you shouldn't eat blueberries; they contain a vast variety of healthy nutrients. What this means is that just one high-quality curcumin capsule delivers more than 25 times the antioxidants as the same number of blueberries.

You've been diagnosed. Now what?

In any case, if you have cancer, you should be working very closely with a trusted oncologist to determine all treatment approaches that are best for you. This includes the use of both modern and traditional options that are scientifically proven to help patients. If your physician is not familiar with the health benefits of curcumin and other complementary and alternative treatment medicines, educate your doctor about it. (See Chapter 12 in this section for a synopsis of this book. We welcome you to print it and give to your doctor.)

Have a meaningful and open discussion about the wealth of scientific evidence that has been published on the anticancer benefits of curcumin individually, and its use in conjunction with conventional cancer treatments.

We think this is the most natural route for conventional doctors to recognize curcumin and the other botanicals we'll be covering in the coming chapters plus their fairly astonishing synergistic effects as a bona fide treatment option for various diseases, including cancer.

In short, if either of us had any type of cancer or any of our loved ones were in that position, we would absolutely use curcumin at all stages of the disease and probably for the rest of everyone's lives.

Most likely it would stop the disease from progressing. There are no serious side effects (sometimes a bit of loose stools at very high doses).

Of course, ideally, we can all use curcumin as a preventive along with other healthy lifestyle habits and the cancer never gets a foothold. But if you or someone you love does get any type of cancer, you definitely should talk to your oncologist about using curcumin. Why not? There is nothing to lose and everything to gain.

In the coming chapters, we'll be examining the ways that curcumin and the other powerhouse natural therapies can exponentially increase one another's arsenals against cancer.

WHAT YOU NEED TO KNOW. . .

Curcumin:

❖ Attacks cancer from several directions ("multi-targeting"), making it potentially even more effective than drugs currently in use in conventional cancer treatment.

❖ Has shown positive effects for virtually every disease for which it has been studied.

❖ Is the most potent anti-inflammatory botanical known to science. It also has one of the highest antioxidant ratings of any food.

❖ Its anticancer properties are unique in the plant world and make it the ideal plant compound to conquer virtually every type of cancer and many chronic diseases.

❖ By itself, or in conjunction with conventional treatment may be a powerful option for patients with various diseases, including cancer.

CHAPTER 7

Andrographis

Andrographis (*Andrographis paniculata*) is a broad-spectrum botanical central to the herbal traditions of several Asian countries. By broad-spectrum, we mean that andrographis has been used for millennia by Traditional Chinese Medicine (TCM) practitioners and Ayurvedic physicians to address a wide range of illnesses from hangovers to cancer and just about anything in between.

In Traditional Chinese medicine, andrographis is classified as a "cold" medicine, helping rid the body of fevers, toxins and heat.

In Ayurvedic medicine, andrographis is similarly considered dry, penetrating and cooling. It is considered kapphapitta, helping remove excess mucous, improving liver function and digestion, and supporting a healthy respiratory tract. Ayurveda is a complex science, so, let it suffice to say that these qualities make it one of the most potent of herbs in the Ayurvedic medicine chest. Only curcumin, ashwagandha and holy basil are more widely used in this indigenous Indian medicine tradition.

In both traditions, the primary purpose of andrographis is to support the immune system, but it is used for many, many more purposes because of its ability to maintain homeostasis or biological balance.

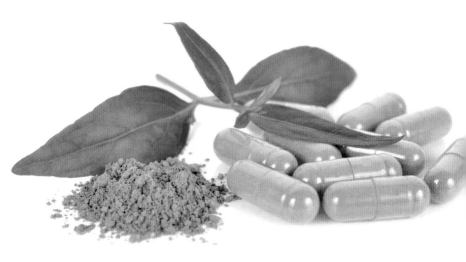

Andrographis is an adaptogen, one of the multi-taskers of the plant world. In the simplest possible terms, adaptogens, like andrographis, are plant medicines that provide your body what it needs to survive.

Many people use adaptogens to prevent or postpone the chronic diseases of aging, recognizing their uncanny ability to fix what's wrong, boost what's right, keep the body in balance and prevent body functions from deteriorating.

Adaptogenic powers like those we see in andrographis have been scientifically validated as effective against chronic inflammation, atherosclerosis (hardening of the arteries), neurodegenerative cognitive impairment (Alzheimer's disease and other forms of dementia), metabolic disorders, diabetes, cancer and a host of other age-related diseases.

As is often the case, the effectiveness of medicines that have been used and revered by indigenous people for millennia is now affirmed by modern science.

In the past couple of years, Dr. Goel and his team have

published six studies on the unique anticancer benefits of andrographis, including a deeper look at the synergistic benefits of andrographis combined with the other botanicals and melatonin featured in this book.

As of this writing, the National Library of Medicine's database returned 1214 published studies on the wide spectrum of health effects of andrographis dating as far back as 1951.

Many of the healing powers of andrographis come from andrographolides, a rare group of diterpenoid lactones, which have strong proven anti-inflammatory, antioxidant and antimicrobial effects. We've already taken a pretty deep dive into the importance of anti-inflammatory and antioxidants in cancer prevention and treatment, so you're probably a step ahead of me in understanding how andrographis can provide protection against cancer and an effective treatment or adjunct treatment if you have the disease.

Andrographis is also a rich source of other nutrients, including well-researched antioxidant flavonoids and polyphenols.

Fights Cancer in Five Ways or More

Andrographis fights cancer in at least five ways (maybe more—new ones are being confirmed frequently!) and has been clinically proven to be effective at slowing, stopping or even eliminating cancer growth in at least eight of the deadliest forms of the disease.

Dr. Goel's most recent research confirms this. His team discovered that not only is andrographis an effective cancer treatment in general, it's even amazingly effective against metastatic gastrointestinal cancers, which are some of those most difficult to treat and therefore the deadliest.

Probably the most impressive overview of the pertinent research on andrographis and cancer comes from an international consortium of 19 scientists that confirmed andrographis' anticancer effects "on almost all types of cell lines" by:

✧ neutralizing free radical damage and inflammation

✧ stopping out-of-control cell lifespans

✧ normalizing immune system response

✧ stopping cells from spreading throughout the body, usually through the bloodstream

✧ killing cancer-causing cells by forcing them to commit suicide and starving them.

Apoptosis

You already know that cell life cycle modulation is an important aspect of understanding and treating cancer. It balances the body's normal cell division process, putting the brakes on the wild cell division that grows cancerous tumors or the sluggish gene signals that turn off the natural balancing system, opening the door to cancer.

Numerous studies have confirmed that andrographis "wakes up" the body's communication pathways to cells and tells them to return to their normal lifespans.

Numerous studies confirm that andrographis induces apoptosis, confirming this process for several types of cancer, including breast, prostate and colon cancer, and melanoma, a deadly type of skin cancer.

Andrographis literally gets the cells' lifespan back on the right track and wipes out tumors.

Korean research on andrographis confirmed the herb's ability to induce apoptosis in gastric cancers and to slow or even stop the growth of tumors through the actions of other anticancer proteins.

Antioxidant

Normal cells have a built-in antioxidant system that declines as we age and becomes less able to neutralize those free radical oxygen molecules, we discussed in the first section of this book. This is the underlying cause of many of the diseases of aging, including cancer, heart disease, diabetes and Alzheimer's.

Andrographis is a "strong antioxidant compound," according to Indian research published in 2014 and confirmed by several later studies, including Polish research published in 2015.

Cell Deterioration

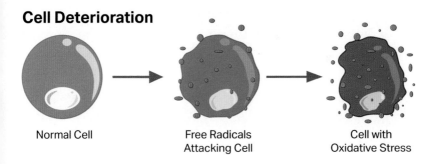

Normal Cell   Free Radicals Attacking Cell   Cell with Oxidative Stress

Immune Booster

As we learned in earlier chapters, andrographis stimulates the immune system, as shown in many studies, largely by activating infection-fighting white blood cells that find and kill bacteria, viruses and other "foreign" substances in the blood.

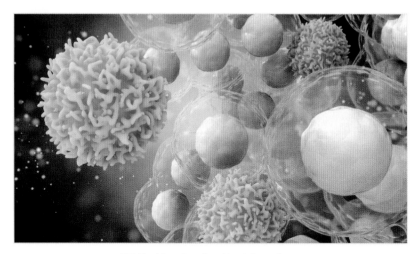

White blood cells attack invaders.

Small doses of andrographolides, natural compounds found in the stems and leaves of the andrographis plant, all contribute to the immune boosting effects of the plant. As you know, in higher doses, andrographis calms down the immune response and inflammation.

Here's some fairly heavy science, for those who love this sort of thing:

As we've already determined, andrographolides are proven anti-inflammatories. This is especially important in a series of cell-signaling proteins called NF-kB that promote cancer in a variety of ways.

NF-κB is present in almost all human cell types and is activated in response to stress, inflammatory substances, free radicals, heavy metals, ultraviolet irradiation and bacterial or viral infections.

NF-kB also has a vital role in protecting against bacterial and viral infections, however it treads a delicate line. Too much

NF-kB is bad because it can turn on genes that tell the cells to divide wildly and stops apoptosis (programmed cell death).

Taiwanese research confirms the value of andrographis in stimulating a very specific anti-inflammatory cell signaling pathway that tells the immune system to fight wild cell division, like we find in cancer.

In the simplest terms, this means that andrographis tells the immune system to control abnormal cell growth.

Angiogenesis

All living beings require nutrients in some form to survive. Cancer cells and cancerous tumors are no different.

Angiogenesis is the process of growing a blood vessel network to nourish a cancerous tumor and allowing it to thrive and grow.

It stands to reason that cutting off that blood supply and oxygen, thus eliminating nutrients, will stop a cancerous tumor from growing and spreading.

Andrographis' ability to cut off the blood supply to tumors is exactly what Chinese researchers were able to confirm with laboratory studies on breast cancer cell lines.

Tumor Suppression

Cell damage means damaged DNA, so cells no longer have the genetic blueprint to reproduce themselves exactly. This results in the formation of tumors, among other problems.

Chinese researchers found that andrographis stops the cycle of melanoma cancer cell growth. Based on past statistics and the fact that the rate of melanoma has been growing for the past 30 years, the American Association for Cancer Research estimated that nearly 100,000 Americans were diagnosed with this potentially deadly form of skin cancer in 2022.

Similar results have been seen in studies of pancreatic cancer cells and in glioblastoma, an aggressive form of brain cancer.

Brand new results confirm that andrographis in combination with oligomeric proanthocyanidins in French grape seed extract also put a halt to tumor growth in animal studies and on test samples grown from tumors of people with colorectal cancer.

Andrographis has also been shown to stop the growth and formation of pancreatic tumor cells and limit the ability of glioblastoma cells to migrate. In each study, andrographis worked along different pathways, showing the versatility of this wonder herb.

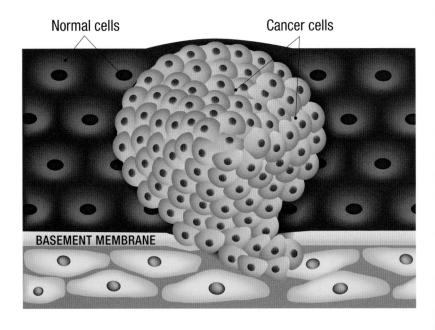

Overall, a recent review showed that andrographolides from andrographis stopped tumor replication in virtually every type of cancer tested and addressed virtually every mechanism, including inflammation, oxidation, cell replication and cancer cell invasion. The authors concluded, "After careful consideration of the relevant evidence, we suggest that andrographolide can be one of the potential agents in the treatment of cancer in the near future."

Enhances Conventional Cancer Therapy

Exciting new research from Dr. Goel's team at the City of Hope Medical Center in California confirms that andrographis significantly improves the effectiveness of conventional chemotherapy treatments. Colorectal cancer is notoriously resistant to conventional chemotherapy drugs, like the commonly used 5-FU. The research confirms that andrographis administered with 5-FU improved responses in people with end-stage colorectal cancer.

Banishes Chemo Brain

Andrographis, the cancer warrior, once again comes to the rescue.

"Chemo brain" is a well-documented side effect of some types of chemotherapy used to treat a wide variety of types of cancer. It's characterized by loss of memory, confusion, difficulty concentrating, searching for words, difficulty learning new skills, brain fog and fatigue.

These are almost precisely the symptoms of various forms of dementia.

The Mayo Clinic adds that chemotherapy is probably not the sole cause of chemo brain and that the psychological and physical stress of a cancer diagnosis can contribute to chemo brain. Radiation and other medications associated with cancer treatment may contribute to memory loss and other brain dysfunction for some cancer patients. Most people with chemo brain improve within six to nine months after treatment has ended, but some have long-term memory loss.

German research published in the journal *Phytomedicine* concluded that chemotherapy drugs in combination with andrographis caused genetic changes that significantly reduced chemo brain. Furthermore, andrographis enhanced the effects of chemotherapy, meaning lower doses of the toxic drug may be effective with fewer side effects.

Chinese researchers confirmed a finding that andrographis works synergistically with a commonly prescribed

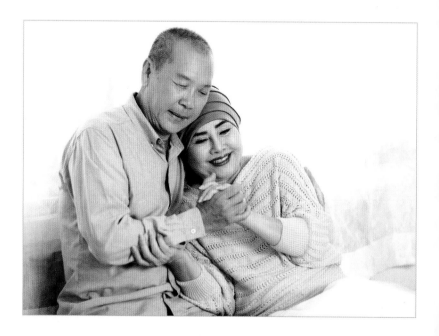

chemotherapy drug for breast cancer (paclitaxel) reducing tumor size by as much as 98%.

One more interesting piece of information from my research team at the City of Hope: Combined with melatonin (that's right, the one you take to help you sleep), andrographis synergistically promotes a wide range of anticancer activities, including autophagy, the process by which the unhealthy cells literally eat themselves, making room for the body to create new, healthy cells.

A note to those who are working with an oncologist: Don't be surprised if your doctor has never heard of andrographis. Don't be surprised if your oncologist says you shouldn't take it. Please turn to the last chapter in this book—it's written in more scientific language aimed directly at your doctors. It's probably not realistic to expect your doctor to read this entire book, but we encourage you to copy those summary pages. It should be very effective at convincing your doctor about the value of andrographis to treat cancer without interfering with other cancer treatments. You might want to copy the reference section as well.

WHAT YOU NEED TO KNOW . . .

Andrographis addresses cancer in at least five ways, possibly more, by:

✤ normalizing immune system response

✤ neutralizing free radical damage and inflammation

✤ stopping out-of-control cell lifespans

✤ stopping cells from spreading throughout the body, usually in the bloodstream

✤ killing cancer-causing cells by forcing them to commit suicide and starving them.

Plus, it enhances the effectiveness of conventional cancer treatment and minimizes its side effects, especially cognitive dysfunction commonly known as "chemo brain."

CHAPTER 8

French Grape Seed Extract

French grape seed comes from the royalty of grapes. Think of French wine and you'll quickly get the idea: There is nothing better!

Our ancestors loved wine fermented from grapes. Today's science has confirmed the health benefits of wine, many of which are derived from the seeds themselves. Concentrating those life-giving and even life-extending benefits into grape seed extract makes French grape seed extract (FGSE) a potent tool that should be part of every household's medicine cabinet.

A major part of French grape seed extract's power comes from substances with the tongue-twisting name, oligomeric proanthocyanidins (OPCs).

Although OPCs are found in many plants, they are concentrated to extraordinary levels in grape seeds, hence their healing power.

OPCs are probably the most potent antioxidants known to science.

You're already well familiar with the power of antioxidants, so it's easy to surmise that French grape seed extract is one of our most important tools in the fight against cancer as well as other chronic diseases.

The Great Neutralizer

OPCs are much more effective than vitamin C and vitamin E and virtually any type of food in neutralizing those destructive free radical oxygen molecules.

The antioxidant levels in French grape seed extract are so high they are quite literally off the scale. The ORAC (oxygen radical absorbance capacity) value of French grape seed extract is so high it is difficult even for modern equipment to accurately measure it. ORAC values are a measure of the free-radical fighting capabilities of a particular food.

Remember back in Chapter 6 when we looked at the high ORAC (antioxidant value) of curcumin? Here's a one-upper: French grape seed extract has an ORAC value of at least 20,000 per gram! That's 25% higher even than the nutrient superstar, curcumin, and higher than any other food!

Foods with high antioxidant power have profound effects on virtually every chronic disease known to science.

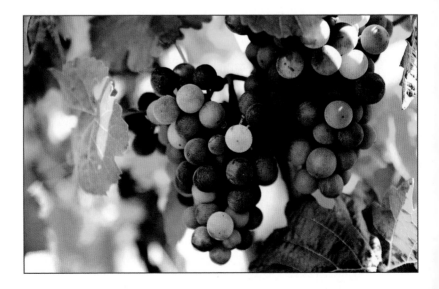

ORAC VALUES (PER 1 GRAM)

French grape seed extract	20,000 or more
Curcumin	15,000 or more
Ginger root	148
Elderberries	147
Cinnamon	131
Acai berries	102
Artichoke	94
Blueberries (raw)	96
Cranberries	90
Basil (dried)	61
Blackberries	59
Red wine (cabernet)	45
Sage (fresh)	32

—Source: U.S. Department of Agriculture

Of course, we are talking about the *right* grape seed extract. In recent years, there have been some cheap products on the market that have little or no value. So-called grape seed extract from China can cost as little as $20 per kilo. In this case, you get what you pay for: Not much.

The best quality grape seed extract comes from tannin-free French OPCs that have a small molecular structure for the best absorbability—and the raw materials cost twenty times as much. It's truly worth it, as you'll see as you progress through this book.

Dr. Goel has done all of his research on a French grape seed extract formulation that he knows is tannin-free and of the best quality.

Combatting Cancer

A substantial body of research has catapulted this unique herbal formulation to the forefront of natural approaches to cancer.

We know that some natural substances—like French grape seed extract and the OPCs in it—can repair genetic damage and tell cancer-preventive genes to wake up and do their jobs or signal genes that are overactive to calm down and behave in a normal manner rather than reproducing wildly. We know OPCs can also eliminate cancer stem cells, the main reason why even "successful" cancer treatment almost always ends with a recurrence.

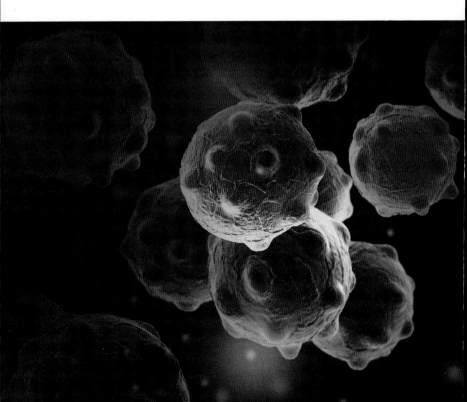

Here's a glimpse of the wide number of ways that French grape seed extract and its OPCs target cancer in a most impressive number of ways. It is scientifically proven to:

✧ Reduce tumor size

✧ Stop cells from becoming cancerous

✧ Relieves inflammation, an underlying cause of cancer

✧ Stop the formation of blood vessels that feed cancerous tumors (angiogenesis)

✧ Signal cancerous cells to commit suicide (apoptosis)

✧ Target cancer stem cells, the major reason why cancers spread (metastasis)

✧ Awaken sleeping genes that stop the growth of cancerous cells or slow down genes that are telling cells to reproduce wildly (epigenetics)

✧ Protect smokers (chemoprevention)

✧ Overcome the body's natural rejection of chemotherapy drugs over time (chemoresistance)

✧ Works synergistically with other natural treatments, including curcumin

✧ Enhance conventional chemotherapy treatments while protecting healthy cells and organs (chemoprotection)

The Research

As you already know, cancer is multifaceted. That means that just one approach will almost never wipe out a particular type of cancer.

And cancer is ever evolving. That means that a treatment that worked last month or even last week, may no longer be effective today for no apparent reason.

Dr. Goel admits that his team's findings over the past five years have surpassed our wildest expectations.

Probably most importantly, using a technique never used before, our team was able to confirm that OPCs stop the mechanism that transforms non- cancerous cells and "normal" cells into specialized and deadly cancer stem cells. These cancer stem cells promote tumor growth, and they can lie dormant in the bloodstream, sometimes for years, only to awaken sometime later, perhaps in the same place or perhaps spreading the cancer to another place in the body. These time bomb stem cells explain why people who have had cancer and have been pronounced "cancer-free" often find themselves with the disease again years later.

This research means that OPCs not only stop the growth of cancerous tumors, but they can also stop cancers from spreading and perhaps they can even prevent cancer altogether.

In addition to telling cancer cells to die when their time comes, the OPCs in French grape seed extract also help kill cancerous tumors by cutting off their blood supply (angiogenesis) and stop the spread of cancer (metastasis) through a wide variety of "pathways," targeting cancer from several directions as is necessary to beat the disease. They even enhance the effectiveness of chemotherapy drugs and radiation therapy commonly used in conventional cancer treatment and help reduce side effects and damage to healthy organs. These discoveries are immensely exciting and prove that low-cost, non-toxic, plant-derived cancer treatments can be extremely effective.

Inhibit the Spread of Cancer Stem Cells

Cancer stem cells have immortality—or near immortality. Think of them as super-cells. As we've learned in earlier chapters, cancer cells do not have a normal lifespan like healthy cells. They live on and on, reproducing in their twisted fashion, creating more cancer cells and larger tumors that can spread throughout the body. They can also send messages to the cancer cells to resist chemotherapy drugs.

These cancer stem cells have an uncanny ability to hide from conventional medicine's diagnostic "radar," lurking in the deepest recesses of the body, appearing to sleep or staying quiet for months, even years, before they awaken and begin to grow again with a vengeance.

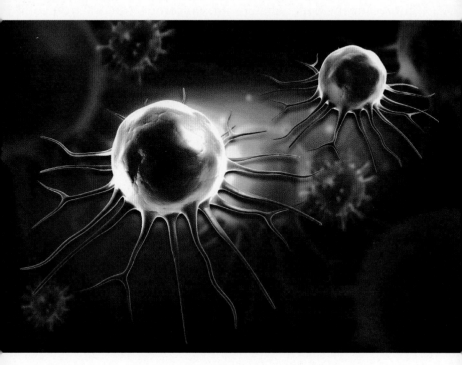

Not only that, but some ordinary cancer cells can also transform themselves into cancer stem cells, increasing their power exponentially.

You'll note we said, "most," but not "all" attempts to kill cancer stem cells have failed. Conventional medicine offers absolutely nothing that can touch them.

Understanding and eliminating cancer stem cells is the cutting edge of cancer research today.

Dr. Goel was honored to lead a creative and brilliant research team at Baylor University's Center for Gastrointestinal Research and the Center for Epigenetics, Cancer Prevention and Cancer Genomics in Dallas until the summer of 2019.

This team was among the first to create cancer organoids for research in botanical treatments for cancer. These are tiny three-dimensional versions of cancerous tumors from our patients and then subjected the organoids to various substances without harming the patients. Think of those organoids as stand-ins identical to the actual tumors.

Organoids are conglomerations of cells, but the unique thing is that they are exact 3D replicas of the cancerous tumors in real human patients. In the past, we have been able to work with laboratory-generated cell lines and animals, but, for ethical reasons, it is extremely complicated to do research on human subjects. Now we can take an exact replica of human tumors outside the patient's body, look directly into them and discover precisely what will work to kill them.

Remember we've said that each patient's cancer is individual and requires unique ways of treating it? These stand-in clones of the actual tumor give us a perfect way to discover the treatments that work as opposed to lab-grown cell cultures or animal experimentation, which may or may not reflect how a given substance might act in humans.

The immensely exciting discovery from our research team is that French grape seed extract is enormously effective in killing cancer stem cells.

Let us repeat that: The OPCs in French grape seed extract *killed* cancer stem cells. Other than curcumin, French grape seed extract is the *only* substance, natural or pharmaceutical, that in our experience stops cancer stem cells from reproducing.

In Dr. Goel's lab, the team exposed those cancer organoids to OPCs and found that in just five days, the presence of cancer in those organoids was dramatically decreased.

These unique studies are the only ones done using human-derived organoids. It proves that botanicals like French grape seed extract can be used for precisely targeted cancer treatments.

Prevents Carcinogenesis

Carcinogenesis is just a fancy term for the beginning of cancer. We are still not really sure what causes normal cells to begin to reproduce wildly and become cancerous. This means cancer cells can begin to clump together and form tumors, like those found in breast, prostate, lung and many other cancers. In some cases, like in leukemia, multiple myeloma and other blood cancers, there are no tumors. The disease is carried in the bloodstream.

If those normal cells continue on the pre-programmed path of life in which they are born, do what they were designed to do and die on schedule, there is no problem. When they somehow deviate from that path, cancer can begin. We don't know exactly how or why this happens, but we do know that lifestyle choices are certainly an important factor. This is especially true with about 90% of colorectal cancer and dietary choices.

So, the ultimate cancer treatment is to prevent it altogether.

OPCs have now been scientifically confirmed to do exactly that.

A study from our team published in 2018 in the journal *Carcinogenesis,* showed that OPCs halted communication in all six known cancer cell-forming pathways. In simple terms, this means that normal cell life cycles cannot be disrupted, so cancer cannot begin. In my mind, this is a good reason for almost everyone to take French grape seed extract on an ongoing basis.

Let us add here that all of the research from our research team has been done on colorectal cancer. There is ample scientific evidence that our results will also apply to many, if not most, other types of cancer, including deadly breast, lung, pancreatic, liver and prostate cancers.

Inhibits Tumorigenesis

Tumorigenesis is the clumping together of abnormal cells to form tumors. Some experts use the term interchangeably with carcinogenesis, we can think of it as the next step in the formation of cancers. In the case of tumor-forming cancer cells, they are different when those rogue cells actually begin to clump together.

In the study published in *Carcinogenesis,* our team showed that OPCs and even French grape seed extract with larger molecules were able to lock down those deviant cells and stop them from clumping together. They were also able to stop those rogue cells from moving around into positions where they can form tumors.

Promotes Apoptosis

While we're on the subject of abnormal cell behavior, let's talk about apoptosis, the process of a natural cellular life cycle. Normal cells are born, perform their function and die on schedule. Some, like skin cells, live only a couple of weeks. Others, like fat cells, hang around for about 8 years while heart muscle cells live about 40 years and brain cells are believed to live as long as 200 years! That raises many fascinating questions for another time.

When cells go rogue and don't die when they should, we have a problem. That's when they become cancerous and form tumors. One of the ways of targeting cancer is to stop that wild cell division and persuade cancerous cells to quite literally commit suicide, returning to their natural life cycles and die as they were genetically programmed to do. Dr. Goel's research shows that process, called apoptosis, is triggered by OPCs in French grape seed extract.

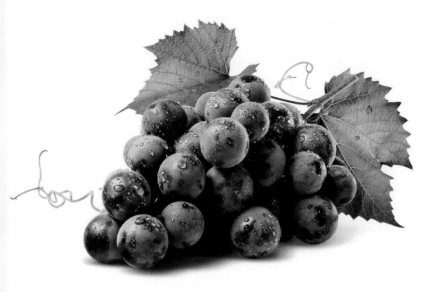

Inhibit Angiogenesis

All living things require nourishment in some form. Plants require sunshine, air and water. Animals (including humans) need food, water, air and sleep.

Cancerous tumors require a blood supply to carry nourishment to the tumors and allow it to grow and thrive. These tumors can actually grow a network of blood vessels to feed them, a process called angiogenesis.

It seems like a simple thing: If you cut off that network of blood vessels, the tumor will die. It does. But it's not just a matter of cutting away blood vessels from a tumor and allowing it to wither away. Think about carcinogenesis, tumorigenesis and apoptosis as I've explained in the previous pages. Then think about all of these things happening at one time. What is needed is something that will hit everything at once.

We do have such a substance: Our research proves that French grape seed extract and the super medicinal OPCs it contains cut off those blood vessels while it is multitasking a slew of other anticancer activities.

There are no pharmaceuticals that have these kind of abilities, largely because conventional anticancer drugs throw those gene-signaling pathways out of balance. They further disrupt homeostasis and require other drugs to try to bring the body back in balance, creating a vicious circle and a downward spiral.

But there is hope and there is an answer!

There are two other botanicals known to have similar properties: curcumin and andrographis. I think the three and others mentioned in this book fit together like puzzle pieces to complete a perfect anticancer picture.

Metastasis

Not only do OPCs reduce tumor growth, but they have also now been scientifically proven to stop the spread of cancer when used with conventional chemotherapy drugs.

Dr. Goel is a scientist, not at all given to hyperbole, but wow. Just Wow! These findings are changing the way doctors treat their patients, even those with late-stage cancers, changing their chances of survival and offering them a vastly improved quality of life.

The One-Two Punch

What if there was another natural treatment that enhanced the already impressive power of French grape seed extract? Then, imagine we put those together and discovered that combined, their power against cancer was multiplied?

That's exactly what my research team found: If you add the OPCs in French grape seed extract to the verified anticancer powers of curcumin, we get a one-two punch against cancer that can't be beat.

In Dr. Goel's study published in *Scientific Reports* in 2018, he found that the botanical combination was doubly effective in preventing carcinogenesis (failures in cell reproduction that start the cancer process) and enhanced other anticancer weapons.

The results were so important that we concluded: "We make a case for the clinical co-administration of curcumin and OPCs as a treatment therapy for patients with colorectal cancer."

He is proud to say that French grape seed extract OPCs join curcumin's elite status. His research shows that hand-in-hand, the anticancer powers of these two botanicals exceeded all expectations.

WHAT YOU NEED TO KNOW . . .

The OPCs in French grape seed extract have unique abilities to target cancer from several ways:

✤ Inhibit the growth and spread of cancer stem cells to keep cancer from recurring.

✤ Prevent carcinogenesis: Stop cells from becoming cancerous at all.

✤ Inhibit tumorigenesis: Stop cancer cells from clumping together and forming cancerous tumors.

✤ Promote apoptosis: Tell wildly reproducing cancer cells to return to their normal life cycles.

✤ Inhibit angiogenesis: Stop tumors from building a blood supply to nourish and sustain them.

✤ Reduce chemoresistance: Make conventional chemotherapy drugs effective.

✤ Inhibit metastasis: Stop cancer from spreading.

French grape seed extract combined with curcumin has anticancer powers that exceed all expectations.

CHAPTER 9

Berberine

Westerners are probably not very familiar with berberine, but it's long been a staple in Ayurvedic and Traditional Chinese Medicine (TCM).

Berberine is an alkaloid compound found in many plants, including Indian and European barberry, Oregon grape, goldenseal, and goldthread. Interestingly, it is also found in abundance in tree turmeric (*Berberis aristate*), a shrub common in India and Nepal. While it is yellow and bitter-tasting, it is not related to *Curcuma longa*, the source of our much-beloved turmeric used as a spice in Indian dishes and curcumin for its vast medicinal powers.

Yet berberine (a/k/a *Berberis vulgaris*) is a botanical with impressive healing properties on its own. It has been used to combat heart disease, high blood pressure, high cholesterol and to regulate blood sugars and treat diabetes for millennia. More recently, it has been validated in Western medicine as an effective preventive and treatment for cancer.

Berberine has long been applauded as an effective treatment for Type 2 diabetes for several reasons, including its effectiveness against belly fat, a major factor in a variety of chronic diseases, including liver disease, non-alcoholic fatty liver disease, liver cancer and several other types of cancer.

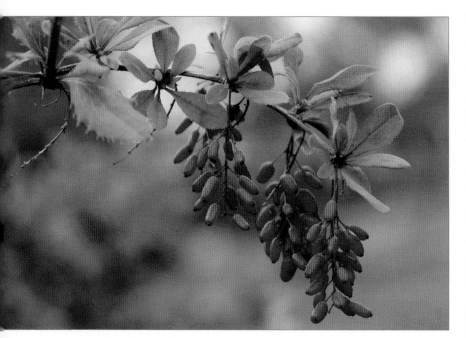

Since we know that obesity is a major risk factor for cancer, among other significant uses, berberine's anti-obesity properties make it an important tool in the arsenal against cancer.

The early use of berberine to treat heart disease and diabetes comes from its impressive antioxidant and anti-inflammatory properties. As you've no doubt surmised from the earlier chapters in this book, those antioxidant and anti-inflammatory properties also translate to the prevention and treatment of many types of cancer.

Effective Against the Deadliest Types of Cancer

Chinese research confirms that berberine combats cancer in many of the ways we've seen in the other natural therapies we are examining in this book by slowing the cellular division that results in malignant tumors, persuading cancerous cells to eat themselves (autophagy—I know, it still sounds a bit gruesome) and persuading them to commit suicide (apoptosis) and slowing cancer spread (metastasis).

A fascinating Chinese human trial confirms that berberine stopped advanced colorectal cancers from recurring and other studies confirm its effectiveness against breast and lung cancers. Other Chinese research shows that berberine effectively treats ulcerative colitis, a well-known cause of gastrointestinal cancers and another confirms effectiveness against liver cancer. Since these are among the deadliest cancers that are the most difficult to treat, this is very welcome news in the treatment and prevention of cancer.

Like the other botanicals we examine in this book, berberine has long been used to fight cancer in TCM. Western science has now confirmed those traditional uses are not only safe, but they are also highly effective.

Numerous studies conclude that berberine is an important component of the anticancer medicine chest for a wide range of reasons.

Major Findings

Here's a litany of the major findings on berberine:

It stops many types of cancerous tumors from forming and growing, including those in the gastrointestinal tract, breast, liver and lungs.

It stops angiogenesis, the blood vessel supply that feeds cancerous tumors.

It triggers apoptosis, the natural life cycle of cancerous cells that causes them to multiply wildly.

In Dr. Goel's experience with people with colorectal cancer, drug resistance becomes a serious problem for virtually all of those with later stage cancers. Overcoming chemoresistance alone will extend their life expectancy and their quality of life. In some cases, berberine actually increased the effectiveness of pharmaceutical chemotherapy drugs, especially those used to treat colorectal and breast cancers.

Berberine also overcomes resistance to chemotherapy drugs, a common issue for later stage cancer patients with all types of cancers.

His most recent study shows that berberine is effective in overcoming resistance to gemcitabine, a chemotherapy drug used to treat many types of cancer, but our work specifically looked at its effectiveness against chemoresistance in pancreatic cancer, one of the deadliest forms of cancer with a dismal survival rate (Only 8 to 10% of pancreatic cancer patients survive five years after diagnosis).

It also has been shown to strengthen body tissues to prevent metastasis, the spread of cancer from one site to another part of the body. For example, breast cancers often migrate to the lungs or the bones.

And...here's something really intriguing: At least one study suggests that berberine helps lengthen telomeres, chemical messengers at the end of each strand of DNA that prevent cellular deterioration due to aging. This could be a major preventive for the genetic malfunctions that eventually weaken the ability of cells to duplicate themselves perfectly as part of their life cycle, opening the way to rogue cells becoming cancerous. That's a huge WOW! Even though it may take a decade or two to really be able to measure the number of cancers that did not happen, it's very exciting news on its own.

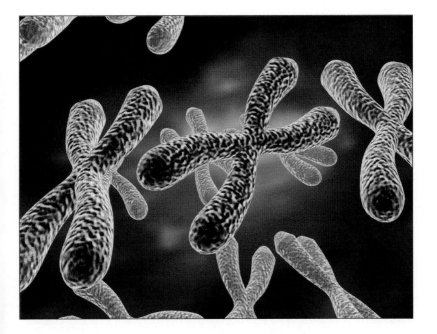

Synergy

Designer drugs may be great, but they cannot compare with the synergy that can take place between the complex botanicals like the ones we are investigating here.

We'll go into this concept in depth in the next chapters, but it's important to note here that when berberine works with other powerful botanicals, its cancer preventive and banishing power is multiplied, sometimes exponentially.

Dr. Goel's research team has recently published two key findings verifying the synergistic effects of berberine when combined with other botanicals.

In the first, they confirmed the "powerful synergistic" anticancer effects from berberine and andrographis, which act together more effectively than each individually, especially in three important ways:

1. To target cancer cells and literally wipe them out before they can clump together to form a tumor.

2. If cancer cells do survive, the berberine/andrographis combo prevents them from clumping together to form tumors.

3. It prevents cancerous cells that have clumped into tumors from duplicating themselves to form more tumors.

We'd almost say, "Who could ask for more?" But there *is* more.

Dr. Goel and his team created a series of complicated tests to determine that a combination of berberine and the oligomeric proanthocyanidins (OPCs) found in French grape seed extract and found they made a truly mind-boggling team to interrupt the chemical signaling pathways that lead to cancer in a wide variety of ways. Remember that all cancers operate on a range of chemical pathways that makes each one unique. If we can better understand that bodily messaging system, we can stop cancers before they start, stop them from growing and stop them from spreading.

Among the ones our team positively confirmed for the berberine/OPC combo is their synergistic message to cause colorectal cancer cells to die. Using cell cultures taken from our patients, we found that the OPCs work like a key to open cancer cells and usher berberine and OPCs into the cancer cells, giving them the message to commit cellular suicide.

Furthermore, a key Chinese study published in *Scientific Reports* in 2016 extols the combination of berberine and curcumin as far more effective than either one used individually to treat breast cancer and that they specifically target at least two cell lines known to cause breast cancer.

Berberine also works with cisplatin, a chemotherapy drug used to treat breast cancer, to dramatically enhance the effectiveness of the drug against apoptosis and metastasis.

Despite all of these impressive findings, standard berberine can still be difficult for the body to absorb and use effectively.

In fact, it's estimated that only about five percent of any given dosage of berberine actually makes it into the bloodstream, so finding a way to enhance absorption is key to the full advantage of its benefits. Look for a product that combines berberine with an ultra-absorbable plant-based delivery system to get the most impact from this botanical.

That's why Dr. Goel used a bioabsorbable berberine from Indian barberry (*Berberis aristata*) in all of his research. He vouches for its effectiveness.

WHAT YOU NEED TO KNOW . . .

Berberine, was broadly used in Ayurvedic and Traditional Chinese Medicine, to treat heart disease and diabetes. It is now enthusiastically endorsed by Western medicine as a powerful preventive and treatment for several of the deadliest types of cancer. It works by:

❖ Stopping DNA deterioration that leads to the birth of cancerous cells.

❖ Stopping cells from clumping together to form tumors.

❖ Promoting apoptosis (programmed death of cancer cells, especially those that are damaged enough to become cancerous).

❖ Promoting autophagy (self-absorption of cancer cells).

❖ Synergistic action with curcumin, andrographis, and French grape seed extract that greatly enhance their anticancer benefits.

CHAPTER 10

Melatonin

M ost of us know about melatonin. Or at least we think we do.

"Melatonin? Isn't that to help you sleep?" you might ask. Very few of us know anything more about this nutrient that offers profound beneficial effects to the entire human organism.

Yes, melatonin does help you sleep. A good night's rest is essential to many areas of general health, including blood sugar control, weight control and yes, immune function.

But melatonin's health benefits go much farther than simply promoting a good night's rest for a wide variety of reasons.

Researchers have long known the link between melatonin and a host of health benefits, especially in older people. For some unexplained reason, our attention has been rivetted on the sleep aspect of melatonin and we've ignored unique and substantial scientific evidence that melatonin does more, so much more.

Primary among melatonin's wonders is immune system enhancement. Numerous studies have confirmed that melatonin strengthens your immune system as well as the large body of scientific evidence that supports its use as an antiviral and antimicrobial in today's challenging world.

Melatonin also has an uncanny ability to help turn back the

clock on the aging process. The process is not yet well understood, but the effects have been documented.

What Exactly Is Melatonin?

Melatonin has been called a hormone and indeed it does have hormone-like properties as a chemical messenger. Technically known as N-acetyl-5-methoxytryptamine, melatonin acts like a hormone in every way except, unlike a hormone, melatonin can actually be extracted from food, including eggs, nuts, tart cherries and goji berries. True hormones are only manufactured by the human body.

In the human body, most melatonin is produced by the pineal, a small pea-sized gland in the center of the brain.

Unlike the plant-based cancer fighters, featured in this book, melatonin is not a botanical. As you'll read in the coming pages, its place in this listing of cancer-fighting powerhouses is well documented and well deserved.

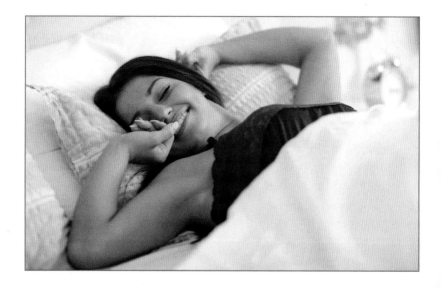

Cancer Prevention

Immune system boosting T-cells are the body's primary cancer fighters. By preventing or slowing the decline of the immune system as we age, melatonin protects your body from cancer by improving the body's ability to identify and eradicate cells that might turn cancerous. There is also research that shows melatonin is particularly effective in preventing hormonally related cancers, including breast and prostate cancer.

For those who have cancer, melatonin should not be taken during chemotherapy, but taken before and after chemotherapy. Melatonin may help protect bone marrow cells from the destructive effects of chemo.

Dr. Goel's former research team at Baylor also found that melatonin overcomes cancer patients' almost inevitable resistance to 5-fluorouracil (5-FU), a chemotherapy drug often used to treat colorectal and other cancers.

As we mentioned in Section 1, modern science now agrees that every cancer is bioindividual. That's scientific language for everyone is different and all cancers are different and, therefore, effective cancer treatment can take a wide range of paths.

Yet, of course, there are some common threads. All cancers:

✧ Are the result of the failure of the system that governs the natural life spans and reproduction of all cells, a process called *apoptosis*.

✧ Create a network of blood vessels to sustain and nourish cancerous cells, a process called *angiogenesis*.

✧ Can spread to other body systems, a process called *metastasis*.

Where does melatonin fit in this picture?

We'll dare say that melatonin's preventive and healing properties are at their peak when it comes to cancer.

Science is discovering more and more that the most effective, cancer-fighting nutrients are those that target the disease from multiple directions.

Melatonin certainly fits that bill.

Apoptosis

What if there was a way to re-establish normal cell growth, cell division and cell death? Or to prevent apoptosis from starting cancerous cellular growth at all?

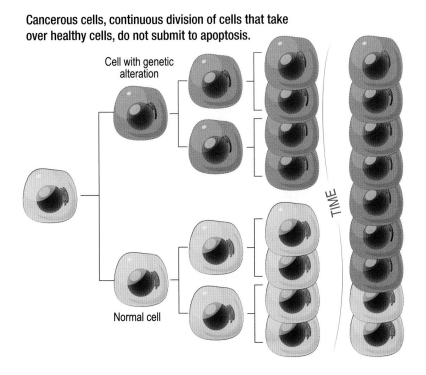

Cancerous cells, continuous division of cells that take over healthy cells, do not submit to apoptosis.

Cell with genetic alteration

Normal cell

TIME

You've probably already guessed that melatonin fits that bill and brings with it many more weapons in the anticancer arsenal.

Italian research confirms that melatonin promotes apoptosis and, because of its antioxidant properties, counteracts the toxicity of chemotherapy agents. This means it increases the effectiveness of chemotherapy, even in patients with advanced lung, breast, gastrointestinal, and head and neck cancers. It also reduces the long term and serious side effects of chemotherapy drugs, including heart problems, nerve damage, anemia, profound fatigue and more.

Research on the underlying reasons why melatonin is effective against cancer in many ways, seems to agree that its antioxidant and anti-inflammatory powers play an important role in cancer prevention and treatment.

Angiogenesis

Like all living things, cancerous tumors need nutrients. You'll remember from earlier chapters that they get these nutrients by creating their own network of blood vessels that feed the tumor and help it grow, a process called angiogenesis.

Melatonin restricts the tumors' ability to feed themselves by cutting off the blood vessel network.

A pivotal 2019 Chinese study says melatonin may be an important anticancer agent because it cuts off the blood to that network, thereby eradicating the tumor's nutrient supply. This seems to be particularly effective against solid tumors like those found in breast and lung cancers, the deadliest cancers in the Western world.

An Iranian study in 2017 also found that melatonin

enhances the ability of chemotherapy agents to stop that blood vessel growth.

Metastasis

Most cancers will metastasize if they are not stopped before they can spread. That is why it is so important to stop cancer at the stages of apoptosis and angiogenesis. But once cancer has spread, it is not the end.

Melatonin has well-documented anti-metastatic properties. An important 2017 study not only confirms that melatonin prevents metastasis, but it also works synergistically with conventional agents against the deadliest cancers.

Epigenetics

Melatonin is produced by the pineal gland in complete darkness. But in the modern world, artificial lighting, television lighting and our various devices emit light late into the hours of darkness when we should be producing melatonin.

That blockage of melatonin production seems to be one of the important epigenetic triggers for the formation of a variety of types of cancerous tumors. Fortunately, research tells us that this epigenetic problem is reversible by increasing available melatonin. This could take place through extended time spent in complete darkness and/or through supplements.

Life Expectancy after Diagnosis

A 2021 University of California Irvine review of scientific evidence for melatonin and cancer concluded that melatonin lengthens the life expectancy of people with a wide variety of types of cancer, regardless of the cancer type or stage, at least partly because it slows the growth of tumors.

The same review of research from the late '90s and early '00s confirms that melatonin improves the effectiveness of all types of conventional cancer treatments, including chemotherapy and radiation and improves the five-year survival rate of even those with difficult and advanced cancers. It was also shown to reduce the pain levels of people with advanced cancers.

The only negative side effect was sleepiness, which isn't surprising considering that melatonin is usually taken to improve sleep.

"There is highly credible evidence that melatonin mitigates cancer at the initiation, progression and metastasis phases," wrote a consortium of University of Texas, Spanish, Mexican and Taiwanese researchers. "What is rather perplexing, however, is the large number of processes by which melatonin reportedly restrains cancer development and growth. These diverse actions suggest that what is being observed are merely epiphenomena (secondary effects) of an underlying, more fundamental action of melatonin that remains to be disclosed."

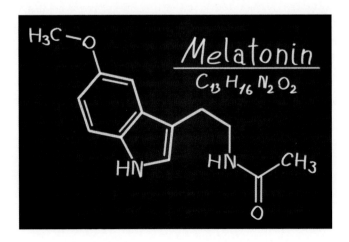

This is scientific lingo for the concept that melatonin is a powerful anticancer agent and researchers don't really know why. Not yet anyway. Stay tuned.

Best of All...

Dr. Goel's research team at City of Hope just published a study that confirms that a combination of melatonin and andrographis act as a synergistic anticancer treatment, especially by inducing apoptosis. In the simplest possible terms, the sooner you are able to return cancerous cells to their normal life spans, the better your chances of complete remission. We'll go further into that kind of synergy in a couple of chapters.

WHAT YOU NEED TO KNOW . . .

Extensive scientific evidence confirms that melatonin is a hormone-like substance produced by the pineal gland that:

✤ Stops the wild cell division that causes cancerous tumors

✤ Stops the formation of blood vessels that feed cancerous tumors

✤ Stops the spread of cancer

✤ Reverses genetic damage caused by lifestyle choices that slow the body's ability to make melatonin

✤ Enhances the effectiveness of conventional chemotherapy drugs

CHAPTER 11

Synergy

From Dr. Goel:

I'm not a superlative kind of guy. I'm a scientist and I admit I'm kind of a geeky one, as you might expect. I spend endless hours in my lab searching out every detail in my research, looking at it from every angle, actively seeking flaws.

That's why I am extremely excited about the potential of the botanicals and melatonin presented in this book to bring about healing in ways that medical science is only just beginning to comprehend.

When we started writing this book, Terry and I thought we'd slowly ease you into all of these ideas about the ways these allied nutrients and melatonin attack cancer:

- ✧ Anti-inflammatory
- ✧ Antioxidant
- ✧ Inducing apoptosis
- ✧ Inhibiting angiogenesis
- ✧ Stopping metastasis
- ✧ Activating autophagy
- ✧ Activating sleeping genes with epigenetics
- ✧ Eliminating cancer stem cells
- ✧ Overcoming chemoresistance
- ✧ Activating chemo-enhancement
- ✧ Protection from tissue damage from chemotherapy and radiation

Our editor warned us that all of these claims might earn me the label of snake oil salesman, readers would doubt my credibility and they'd be unlikely to read the chapters that document the scientific proof of the power of curcumin, andrographis, French grape seed extract, berberine and melatonin against cancer.

Now that you've read the explanations and the science, when you add them all up, there is no doubt at all that they work and often work synergistically to enhance the already substantial healing powers to attack cancer from many angles without serious side effects.

> *Individually, these ingredients work like no other substances known to science, whether natural or pharmaceutical, to prevent, attack and overcome cancer. When we add these complementary nutrients together, the synergistic benefits are nothing short of amazing.*

What Is Synergy?

You may have heard the word, but what exactly is synergy and how does it apply to the treatment and prevention of cancer?

Synergy is defined as a combination of factors that result in something greater than the sum of the parts.

It's sort of like 2 + 2 = 5 or maybe even 2 + 2 = 10. That's new math for sure! It's directly applicable to curcumin and its natural companions we're talking about in this book.

To make all of this simple: All of these nutrients work together in a wide and complex network of ways to combat and prevent cancer with a high rate of success, even in people with advanced cancers.

Remember that in earlier chapters we talked about the

multiple pathways that can cause cells to go rogue and become cancerous?

When we combine these botanical super plants and/or melatonin in any number of ways, we address those pathways in ways never before understood by modern science.

Can you take them all together? Absolutely! Or you can tailor them to your individual needs and risks.

Of course, you should do this under the care of an integrative medical practitioner who knows about the properties of these nutrients or at least is willing to learn about them. You might want to donate a copy of this book to your practitioner's education!

If you have cancer, it is probably not necessary for you to take all of these botanicals and melatonin. An excellent healthcare practitioner will help you find the right combination depending on the type of cancer you have, what stage (how far it has progressed), your age and gender and other medical factors, such as obesity, pre-existing heart disease and/or diabetes.

So now we need to take a look at the best ways to incorporate these super nutrients into your preventive regimen and, if you've been diagnosed with cancer, we'll look at formulations that target cancer in a variety of ways.

Curcumin Is Key

Let us first say that we firmly believe curcumin is the foundation of any and all cancer prevention and cancer treatment regimens.

If you have been diagnosed with any type of cancer or you have any of the risk factors we discussed in earlier chapters, PLEASE start taking curcumin today.

Dosages and strengths vary depending on your state of health, but here's a quick reminder:

Curcumin is not very absorbable or bioavailable in general.

Curcumin: The Star of Our Show

Curcumin should be the central focus for anyone with cancer or for anyone at high risk for cancer. We know of no negative side effects of any of the nutrients mentioned in this book when they are taken at the recommended dosages. Higher dosages could be warranted for those with advanced cancers, but you should always work with a caring integrative practitioner before increasing dosage beyond the label recommendations

Adding in any of the allied anticancer nutrients is your choice, but we think andrographis, French grape seed extract, melatonin and berberine are all well worth your consideration.

Bioavailability vs. Bioactivity

Many studies emphasize curcumin's low *bioavailability.* That means that the human body can't easily access the nutrients and health benefits it offers. In simple terms, we're talking about absorption into the blood through the digestive tract.

Despite low levels of high-quality curcumin supplements in the blood of people taking it, thousands of studies confirm its *bioactivity*—its effectiveness in treating and preventing disease, including cancer. This suggests curcumin doesn't work like an aspirin—you can't swallow it with a glass of water and it takes care of the problem. That means it *must* work in another way. What we know for sure is that it *does* work!

Low blood levels of curcumin are not at all a deal breaker.

Let's explore a little painless biochemistry first.

There are four basic reasons why curcumin doesn't show up in large amounts in the bloodstream:

1. Low water solubility

2. Poor absorption through the digestive tract

3. Metabolic conversion of the curcumin after consuming it, making it hard to detect in blood

4. Binding of curcumin to cellular proteins in various body tissues, resulting in less curcumin circulating in the bloodstream

Low Water Solubility

Low water solubility is not a problem for digestive cancers, particularly colorectal cancer, since curcumin is absorbed along the digestive tract in exactly the way any food is absorbed. Water is not necessary for this action.

Curcumin is fat soluble. When it is taken by mouth, curcumin is detectable in the brain, which may in part explain its effectiveness in preventing and treating brain diseases.

Other new research suggests that the parent curcumin molecule may not be the most important part here. It's a case of the child becoming more powerful than the parent. Research shows us that when curcumin is processed by the liver, it is broken down into many components, each of which has its own benefits. Some of those metabolites of curcumin have their own antitumor and anti-inflammatory effects, adding to their effectiveness against cancer and other diseases.

It's also possible that many of curcumin's components have already been used by the body (metabolized) by the time blood is tested to determine if they are still present. In addition, some of them are known to be water soluble and they will show up in blood tests, but they are no longer recognizable as curcumin.

Best Bioavailability

We're not going to recommend specific products here, but there is one formulation of curcumin that I have used in my research because it is much more bioavailable than ordinary curcumin supplements, which are only 50 to 60% absorbed by weight. This means the curcumin's absorption can be seen in blood tests.

The curcumin I use in my research is blended with essential oils from turmeric based on the centuries-old Ayurveda system, so the product is all natural. It has been shown to have 7 to 10 times higher bioavailability and research shows it is retained longer in the circulatory system than standard curcumin. There are curcumin products that claim higher bioavailability, but their fatty coating is synthetic. Additionally, it is very important to note that turmeric essential oil contains turmerones, which are themselves anticancer and have been shown to boost the activity of curcumin.

One study shows that this curcumin has a double peak action. It shows up in the bloodstream of human subjects within an hour and drops for a short period of time, then rises again 4.5 hours later and remains detectable in the blood after eight hours. That means not only is it absorbed, it remains in the system much longer than other curcumin supplements, which typically dissipate within a little more than two hours.

This formulation is clearly superior because it is easily absorbed and contains compounds (turmerones) that boost curcumin's effectiveness. I have used it in all of my research because several well-designed studies confirm that this curcumin provides measurable health benefits. It is also one of the most clinically studied, enhanced absorption curcumin products.

Curcumin is often combined with boswellia (also known as frankincense), for increased anti-inflammatory effects.

What Works with What

My team has published more than 30 studies on the effectiveness of various botanicals against cancer. While most of my research focuses on colorectal cancer, we have confidence that our results also apply to many other types of cancer, many of them the deadliest ones.

I can say with confidence that if you or a loved one is battling cancer or is at high risk for any type of cancer, you and your health care provider should seriously consider these combinations.

In addition to the considerable individual anticancer benefits of curcumin, andrographis, French Grape Seed Extract, berberine and melatonin, my research confirms the following:

✧ **Curcumin** and the oligomeric proanthocyanidins (OPCs) in **French grape seed extract (FGSE)** combine to target even larger numbers of cancer pathways than either one individually.

✧ **Berberine** and the oligomeric proanthocyanidins in **French grape seed extract** work together as a formidable combination through a wide range of signaling pathways that approach cancer with exactly the multi-targeted approach that we know is effective.

⬧ **Berberine** and **andrographis** combined to target cancer cells before they can clump together to form a tumor, if tumors have already formed, to prevent tumor growth and tumor spread.

⬧ **Melatonin** and **andrographis** promote autophagy (cancerous cells eating themselves and stopping cancer growth).

⬧ **Andrographis** and **French grape seed extract** combine to slow cancer cell growth, stop cancer cells from clumping together to form tumors and persuade cells to die when their life cycle is done rather than becoming cancerous.

We are able to confirm the effects of these powerful botanicals and melatonin against very individual cancers by creating organelles or clumps of actual cancer cells taken from patients with colorectal cancers, some of them with very advanced cases and grown in our lab. This way, we are looking at actual bio-individual cancers rather than cases that exist only in theory. This helps us understand the commonalities and uniqueness of cancers that puts us at the cutting edge of science today.

Other research has confirmed these findings and expanded on them.

⬧ Iranian research shows that **curcumin** and **berberine** combine synergistically to improve the effectiveness of chemotherapy for breast cancer.

⬧ Similar results have been found for the combo against gastric cancers.

⬧ A combination of curcumin+berberine has also been shown to promote apoptosis and autophagy.

This is such a new area of research that I have no doubt that in the near future we will have much more research confirming the synergistic effects of these plant-based and natural approaches as well as many others.

Should you consider three or four or more of these natural powerhouses against cancer? Research will take us there very soon, but I can say for now that these approaches are inexpensive in comparison to the costs of pharmaceutical, surgical and radiation treatments for cancer. We know they are highly effective and, perhaps most of all, they have few if any side effects compared to the terrible side effects of chemotherapy that can actually be the cause of death rather than the cancer itself.

What to Look for When You're Looking for the Right Supplements

I'm the first to agree with you that there are overwhelming numbers of products on the market, and it can be extremely difficult to choose one that will be effective and not break your budget.

How can you navigate those choppy waters?

Here's what I've discovered in my decades of research on natural products:

◇ The cheapest product is usually not the best.

◇ Your supplement should be GMO free.

◇ Look for products manufactured in a cGMP (current good manufacturing practices) compliant facility.

◇ Avoid fillers like sugar, salt, yeast, wheat, gluten, corn, soy, dairy products, artificial coloring, artificial flavoring or preservatives.

Patients always ask me what brands I recommend. That's such an important question because there are so many brands on the market. Some are basically worthless, while there are other high-quality brands you can always depend on. I recommend visiting your local health food store for help identifying products of the highest and most consistent quality in the industry, and which are sustainably produced and standardized.

YOUR GUIDE TO THE HIGHEST QUALITY PRODUCTS

- ✤ Curcumin with turmeric essential oil

- ✤ Andrographis standardized to andrographolides

- ✤ French grape seed extract

- ✤ Melatonin

- ✤ Berberine

I understand that this combination may be a bit pricey for some people. Of course, this is just a tiny fraction of the cost of chemo and radiation. Nevertheless, if you've been diagnosed with cancer and your budget simply won't accommodate the entire regimen and you must make some choices, please opt for curcumin and andrographis for the best bang for your buck. The science confirming their effectiveness is impressive.

CONCLUSION

Anyone who has had cancer knows that doctors are extremely reluctant to proclaim that a patient is "cured." Yet that is the word every patient and every family member wants to hear.

Yes, we know that doctors will say a patient is in remission or even long-term remission after 5 or 10 years have passed cancer-free. However, many doctors and patients feel the shadow of cancer may again rise up. They are correct—sometimes it does.

Yet, I am boldly saying today that we are approaching the time when a supplement cocktail like the combination we have been examining in this book will enable us to actually prevent cancer and possibly cure patients, even some with late-stage cancers. More research is needed, but their promise in dealing with cancer has already been repeatedly validated.

Right now, we can say with confidence that curcumin and andrographis, and their well-studied allies, enable people with almost every kind of cancer to live longer, sometimes much longer, than was originally projected when they were diagnosed.

Cancer treatment is a very personal choice.

We encourage people with cancer to discuss this book with their practitioners and decide, after weighing all the evidence, that curcumin and andrographis are right for them.

Whether you decide to pursue active mainstream treatment or decide to avoid these treatments or pursue a combination of both, curcumin, andrographis, French grape seed extract, melatonin and berberine can play an important role in your health.

And those who choose them in combination with conventional treatments that usually include chemotherapy and radiation can rest assured that they are enhancing the effectiveness of those therapies while protecting healthy tissues from the side effects of those treatments that can ravage the body.

Most important for those who are healthy and wish to remain healthy (who doesn't?), these five super nutrients offer effective prevention, not only against almost all types of cancer, but also against other debilitating diseases, including diabetes, heart disease, obesity, Alzheimer's, depression, digestive disorders, arthritis and joint pain.

Curcumin and andrographis are at the heart of a protocol that can prevent you from tipping the scales toward these diseases due to epigenetic, environmental and lifestyle causes. If you have been diagnosed and treated for cancer, I strongly urge you to take curcumin and andrographis and continue taking them every day for the rest of your life to prevent cancer stem cells from bringing about a recurrence.

Consider adding its partners—like French grape seed extract, berberine and melatonin—that can expand your health and vitality and even prevent cancer from becoming a concern at all.

CHAPTER 12

The Right Combo

From Terry Lemerond:

I'm the first to agree with you that there are overwhelming numbers of these products on the market. It can be extremely difficult to choose the ones that will be effective and not break your budget.

How can you navigate those choppy waters?

Here's what both Dr. Goel and I have discovered in our decades of research on natural products:

✧ The cheapest product is usually not the best. Many have fillers, ineffective ingredients and sometimes even toxic additions.

✧ Your supplement should be GMO free.

✧ Look for products manufactured in a cGMP (current good manufacturing practices) compliant facility.

✧ Avoid fillers like sugar, salt, yeast, wheat, gluten, corn, soy, dairy products, artificial coloring, artificial flavoring or preservatives.

At the risk of being repetitious, Dr. Goel and I are frequently asked what brands we recommend. That's such an important question because there are so many brands on the market. Some are basically worthless, while there are other high-quality brands you can always depend on. I recommend visiting your local health food store and asking for their assistance in identifying products of the highest and most consistent quality in the industry, and which are sustainably produced and standardized.

YOUR GUIDE TO THE HIGHEST QUALITY PRODUCTS

❖ Curcumin with proven bioavailability with turmeric essential oil: 750 mg 2–3 softgel capsules daily for those who have been diagnosed with cancer

❖ Andrographis: 400 mg standardized at 20% yielding 80 mg of andrographolides, 400 mg 2–3 times daily

❖ French grape seed extract: tannin free, 400 mg soft-gel capsules, 2–3 daily

❖ Melatonin: sustained released 10–20 mg as close to sunset as you can

❖ Berberine with gamma-cyclodextrin: 250–500 mg

I understand that this combination may be a bit pricey for some people. Of course, this is just a tiny fraction of the cost of chemo and radiation. Nevertheless, if you've been diagnosed with cancer and your budget simply won't accommodate the entire regimen and you must make some choices, please opt for curcumin and andrographis for the best bang for your buck. The science confirming their effectiveness is impressive.

CONCLUSION

From both of us:

Anyone who has had cancer knows that doctors are extremely reluctant to proclaim that a patient is "cured." Yet that is the word every patient and every family member wants to hear.

Yes, we know that doctors will say a patient is in remission or even long-term remission after 5 or 10 years have passed cancer-free. However, many doctors and patients feel the shadow of cancer may again rise up. They are correct—sometimes it does.

Yet, we are boldly saying today that we are approaching the time when a supplement cocktail like the combination we have been examining in this book will enable us to actually prevent cancer and possibly cure patients, even some with late-stage cancers. More research is needed, but their promise in dealing with cancer has already been repeatedly validated.

Right now, we can say with confidence that curcumin and andrographis, and their well-studied allies, enable people with almost every kind of cancer to live longer, sometimes much longer, than was originally projected when they were diagnosed.

Cancer treatment is a very personal choice.

We encourage people with cancer to discuss this book with their practitioners and decide, after weighing all the evidence, that curcumin and andrographis are right for them.

Whether you decide to pursue active mainstream treatment or decide to avoid these treatments—or pursue a combination of conventional and integrative treatments—curcumin, andrographis, French grape seed extract, melatonin and berberine can play an important role in your health.

And those who choose them in combination with conventional treatments that usually include chemotherapy and radiation can rest assured that they are enhancing the effectiveness of those therapies while protecting healthy tissues from the side effects of those treatments that can ravage the body.

Most important for those who are healthy and wish to remain healthy (who doesn't?), these five super nutrients offer effective prevention, not only against almost all types of cancer, but also against other debilitating diseases, including diabetes, heart disease, obesity, Alzheimer's, depression, digestive disorders, arthritis and joint pain.

Curcumin and andrographis are at the heart of a protocol that can prevent you from tipping the scales toward these diseases due to epigenetic, environmental and lifestyle causes. If you have been diagnosed and treated for cancer, we strongly urge you to take curcumin and andrographis and continue taking them every day for the rest of your life to prevent cancer stem cells from bringing about a recurrence.

Consider taking their partners—like French grape seed extract, berberine and melatonin—that can expand your health and vitality and even prevent cancer from becoming a concern at all.

CHAPTER 13

Message to Healthcare Practitioners

From Ajay Goel, Ph.D., AGAF, *City of Hope Professor and Chair, Department of Molecular Diagnostics and Experimental Therapeutics; Associate Director of Basic Science, Comprehensive Cancer Center (formerly Baylor University's Center for Gastrointestinal Research and the Center for Epigenetics, Cancer Prevention and Cancer Genomics)*

Most authors are very protective of their work and prohibit copying and distributing book contents unless they are sold or pay a fee.

This section of this book is very different. This information is so important that I want to see it distributed far and wide. At least as far as this chapter goes, I am unconcerned about copyright.

I also know that doctors and other healthcare practitioners are very busy. They are very unlikely to read an entire book, even though, like this book, it may contain some information that could save the lives or help improve the quality of life of their patients. I understand that doctors are frequently skeptical about natural formulations and, if they haven't conducted their own research investigations on a subject, they are inclined to steer their patients away from them, even though these formulations might be lifesaving.

I've created this very short chapter, a synopsis of the most important elements of this book. I encourage you to copy it freely. Give it to your doctor or other healthcare practitioner and encourage them to spend ten minutes reading and digesting these short pages.

Dear Doctor,

Your patient has given you a copy of this chapter with my blessings and permission. My publisher and I have given it to the public domain so that the vital information it contains on the value of curcumin, other significant botanicals and melatonin in prevention and treatment of a wide range of cancers can be broadly circulated.

In this book, I am specifically examining the individual and synergistic properties of curcumin (*Curcuma longa*), andrographis (*Andrographis paniculata)*, berberine (*Berberis vulgaris*), oligomeric proanthocyanidins (from French grape seed extract—*Vitis vinifera)* and melatonin.

I have spent more than 20 years researching the preventive and treatment properties of botanicals in my previous tenure at Baylor University and my current tenure at the City of Hope.

My team and I have published more than 30 studies on the subject matter of this book, primarily on curcumin (*Curcuma longa*). I've published more than 400 studies on various aspects of health and cancer, including numerous studies emphasizing the health benefits of complementary and alternative medicine and treatments based on Traditional Chinese Medicine and Ayurvedic tradition.

I am convinced that curcumin can offer broad benefits to prevent, treat and perhaps even cure a wide variety of types of cancers with virtually no side effects.

Most of my research is on botanicals and colorectal cancer. My team and I have based our research on organelles obtained from the tissue biopsies of actual cancer patients. I submit that findings based on colorectal cancer patients are applicable to patients with many types of cancers.

Of course, I am not the only researcher investigating the benefits of plant-based, natural and integrative treatments for cancer. More than 7,000 studies have been published on curcumin's anticancer activity alone, showing benefits dating back to 1983 but the vast majority in the past 20 years. Add in andrographis, oligomeric proanthocyanidins, berberine and melatonin and you'll have a total of nearly 12,000 studies listed in the National Library of Medicine's database. Many of these studies are well constructed and highlight the scientific merit for this natural medicine.

These studies are definitive. They verify the anticancer properties of every single one of these botanicals and melatonin that show individually they target carcinogenesis and metastasis and target the spread of cancer stem cells in ways that are through a broad variety of pathways. Many of them also modulate microRNAs, an especially significant finding in light of today's proliferation of toxic environmental exposures. Several verify synergistic qualities of two or more of these components as well.

I'm sure you are aware of precision medicine and the value of genetics, environment and lifestyle in order to select treatment that will work best for your patients. You can tailor a cocktail of these ingredients based on individual needs and profile. In my mind, this is the single most valuable development in cancer treatment in recent years.

I'm sure you are also aware that the vast majority of pharmaceuticals in common use today were developed from plant sources. I submit to you that many of these pharmaceuticals used in cancer treatment eventually fail and often cause dire side effects that may actually kill the patient. This is precisely because developers of these pharmaceuticals have neglected to recognize the synergistic effects of the vast array of thousands of elements that comprise just one single plant molecule. That is the source of my focus on botanicals and other natural substances.

In brief, this is what we've learned from verifiable results about these botanicals and melatonin, and their effects on cancer cells and the genes that govern them:

Anticancer actions:

- ✧ Anti-inflammatory
- ✧ Antioxidant
- ✧ Antimicrobial
- ✧ Antitumor
- ✧ Chemoprevention

- ✧ Chemosensitivity
- ✧ Chemoprotective
- ✧ Immunostimulant
- ✧ Tumor suppressive

They induce:

- ✧ Apoptosis

- ✧ Autophagy

They inhibit:

✧ Angiogenesis

✧ Stem cell migration

✧ Carcinogenesis

✧ Tumorogenesis

✧ Metastasis

They overcome:

✧ Chemoresistance

They also:

✧ Enhance effectiveness of several chemotherapy protocols

✧ Are chemoprotective/radioenhancing

✧ Modulate or eliminate "chemo brain"

✧ Are affordable

✧ Have no serious side effects or co-morbidities

✧ Enhance quality of life for cancer patients

✧ Extend lifespan of patients with end-stage cancers

Patients always ask me what brands I recommend. That's such an important question because there are so many brands on the market. Some are basically worthless, while there are other high-quality brands you can always depend on. I seek out products from reputable companies to use in all of my research because these products are of the highest and most consistent quality in the industry and are sustainably produced and standardized.

YOUR GUIDE TO THE
HIGHEST QUALITY PRODUCTS

There are many formulations of these products on the market, some much more bioavailable than others. For the sake of consistency, I have used the following formulations of these botanicals and melatonin in my research, so I can vouch for their safety, efficacy and quality:

❖ Curcumin with turmeric essential oil

❖ Andrographis standardized to andrographolides

❖ French grape seed extract (tannin free)

❖ Melatonin

❖ Berberine

In closing, I can only implore you to make an effort to learn more about the value of these treatment options and to consider incorporating them in your treatment plan for your patients.

—Ajay Goel, Ph.D., AGAF

References

Published studies by Dr. Goel on these subjects:

Curcumin

Weng W, Goel A. Curcumin and colorectal cancer: an update and current perspective on this natural medicine. *Semin Cancer Biol.* 2022 May;80:73-86.

Jung G, Goel A et al. Epigenetics of colorectal cancer: biomarker and therapeutic potential. *Nat Rev Gastroenterol Hepatol.* 2020 Feb;17(2):111-130.

Yoshida K, Goel A et al. Curcumin sensitizes pancreatic cancer cells to gemcitabine by attenuating PRC2 subunit EZH2, and the lncRNA PVT1 expression. *Carcinogenesis.* 2017 Oct 1;38(10):1036-1046.

Toden S, Goel A et al. Curcumin mediates chemosensitization to 5-fluorouracil through miRNA-induced suppression of epithelial-to-mesenchymal transition in chemoresistant colorectal cancer. *Carcinogenesis.* 2015 Mar;36(3):355-67.

Shakibaei M. Goel A et al. Curcumin potentiates antitumor activity of 5-fluorouracil in a 3D alginate tumor microenvironment of colorectal cancer. *BMC Cancer.* 2015 Apr 10;15:250.

Sanmukhani J, Satodia V, Goel A et al. Efficacy and safety of curcumin in major depressive disorder: a randomized controlled trial. *Phytother Res.* 2014 Apr;28(4):579-85.

C Buhrmann, Goel A et al. Curcumin suppresses crosstalk between colon cancer stem cells and stromal fibroblasts in the tumor microenvironment: potential role of EMT. *PLoS One.* 2014 Sep 19;9(9):e107514.

Shakibaei M, Goel A et al. Curcumin chemosensitizes 5-fluorouracil resistant MMR-deficient human colon cancer cells in high density cultures. *PLoS One.* 2014 Jan 3;9(1):e85397.

Shakibaei M, Goel A et al. Curcumin enhances the effect of chemotherapy against colorectal cancer cells by inhibition of NF-κB and Src protein kinase signaling pathways. *PLoS One.* 2013;8(2):e57218.

Link A, Balaguer F, Goel A et al. Curcumin modulates DNA methylation in colorectal cancer cells. *PLoS One.* 2013;8(2):e57709.

Chandran B, Goel A. A randomized, pilot study to assess the efficacy and safety of curcumin in patients with active rheumatoid arthritis. *Phytother Res.* 2012 Nov;26(11):1719-25.

Reuter S, Goel A et al. Epigenetic changes induced by curcumin and other natural compounds. *Genes Nutr.* 2011 May;6(2):93-108.

Goel A, Aggarwal BB. Curcumin, the golden spice from Indian saffron, is a chemosensitizer and radiosensitizer for tumors and chemoprotector and radioprotector for normal organs. *Nutr Cancer.* 2010;62(7):919-30.

Goel A, Jhurani S. Aggarwal BB. Multi-targeted therapy by curcumin: how spicy is it? *Mol Nutr Food Res.* 2008 Sep;52(9):1010-30.

Goel A, Kunnumakkara AB, Aggarwal BB. Curcumin as "Curecumin": from kitchen to clinic. *Biochem Pharmacol.* 2008 Feb 15;75(4):787-809.

Andrographis

Zhao Y, Goel A et al. A combined treatment with melatonin and andrographis promotes autophagy and anticancer activity in colorectal cancer. *Carcinogenesis.* 2022 Apr 25;43(3):217-230.

Zhao Y, Goel A et al. A Combined Treatment with Berberine and Andrographis Exhibits Enhanced Anti-Cancer Activity through Suppression of DNA Replication in Colorectal Cancer. *Pharmaceuticals (Basel).* 2022 Feb 22;5(3):262.

Ma R, Goel A et al. Antitumor effects of Andrographis via ferroptosis-associated genes in gastric cancer. *Oncol Lett.* 2021 Jul;22(1):523.

Ma R, Shimura, Goel A et al. Antitumor effects of Andrographis via ferroptosis-associated genes in gastric cancer. *Oncol Lett.* 2021 Jul;22(1):523.

Zhao Y, Wang C, Goel A. Andrographis overcomes 5-fluorouracil-associated chemoresistance through inhibition of DKK1 in colorectal cancer. *Carcinogenesis.* 2021 Jun 21;42(6):814-825.

Shimura T, Goel A et al. Enhanced anti-cancer activity of andrographis with oligomeric proanthocyanidins through activation of metabolic and ferroptosis pathways in colorectal cancer. *Sci Rep.* 2021 Apr 6;11(1):7548.

Sharma P, Goel A et al. Andrographis-mediated chemosensitization through activation of ferroptosis and suppression of β-catenin/Wnt-signaling pathways in colorectal cancer. *Carcinogenesis.* 2020 Oct 15;41(10):1385-1394.

Ravindranathan P, Goel A et al. A combination of curcumin and oligomeric proanthocyanidins offer superior anti-tumorigenic properties in colorectal cancer. *Sci Rep.* 2018 Sep 14;8(1):13869.

French Grape Seed Extract

Ravindranathan P, Goel A et al. Oligomeric proanthocyanidins (OPCs) from grape seed extract suppress the activity of ABC transporters in overcoming chemoresistance in colorectal cancer cells. *Carcinogenesis.* 2019 May 14;40(3):412-421.

Toden S, Goel A et al. Oligomeric proanthocyanidins (OPCs) target cancer stem-like cells and suppress tumor organoid formation in colorectal cancer. *Sci Rep.* 2018 Feb 20;8(1):3335.

Melatonin

Sakatani A, Goel A et al. Melatonin-mediated downregulation of thymidylate synthase as a novel mechanism for overcoming 5-fluorouracil associated chemoresistance in colorectal cancer cells. *Carcinogenesis.* 2019 May 14;40(3):422-431

Berberine

Okuno K, Caiming X, Goel A et al. Berberine overcomes gemcitabine-associated chemoresistance through regulation of Rap1/PI3K-Akt signaling in pancreatic ductal adenocarcinoma. *Pharmaceuticals* (Basel). 2022 Sep 28;15(10):1199. doi: 10.3390/ph15101199.

Boswellia

Takahasi M, Goel A et al. Boswellic acid exerts antitumor effects in colorectal cancer cells by modulating expression of the let-7 and miR-200 microRNA family. *Carcinogenesis.* 2012 Dec;33(12):2441-9.

Synergistic Combinations

Okuno K, Garg R, Goel A et al. berberine and oligomeric proanthocyanidins exhibit synergistic efficacy through regulation of PI3K-Akt signaling pathway in colorectal cancer. *Front Oncol.* 2022 May 4;12:855860.

Zhao Y, Wang C, Goel A. A combined treatment with melatonin and andrographis promotes autophagy and anticancer activity in colorectal cancer. *Carcinogenesis.* 2022 Apr 25;43(3):217-230.

Zhao Y, Roy S, Goel A et al. A combined treatment with berberine and andrographis exhibits enhanced anti-cancer activity through suppression of DNA replication in colorectal cancer. *Pharmaceuticals (Basel).* 2022 Feb 22;15(3):262.

Shimura T, Sharma P, Goel A et al. Enhanced anti-cancer activity of andrographis with oligomeric proanthocyanidins through activation of metabolic and ferroptosis pathways in colorectal cancer. *Sci Rep.* 2021 Apr 6;11(1):7548.

Ravindranathan P, Pasham D, Goel A. Oligomeric proanthocyanidins (OPCs) from grape seed extract suppress the activity of ABC transporters in overcoming chemoresistance in colorectal cancer cells. *Carcinogenesis.* 2019 May 14;40(3):412-421. doi: 10.1093/carcin/bgy184.

Sakatani A, Soniohara F, Goel A. Melatonin-mediated downregulation of thymidylate synthase as a novel mechanism for overcoming 5-fluorouracil associated chemoresistance in colorectal cancer cells. *Carcinogenesis.* 2019 May 14;40(3):422-431.

Ravindranathan, P, Goel A et al. A combination of curcumin and oligomeric proanthocyanidins offer superior anti-tumorigenic properties in colorectal cancer. *Sci Rep.* 2018 Sep 14;8(1):13869.

Ravindranathan P, Pasham D Goel A et al. Mechanistic insights into anticancer properties of oligomeric proanthocyanidins from grape seeds in colorectal cancer. *Carcinogenesis.* 2018 May 28;39(6):767-777.

Toden S, Ravindranathan P, Goel A et al. Oligomeric proanthocyanidins (OPCs) target cancer stem-like cells and suppress tumor organoid formation in colorectal cancer. *Sci Rep.* 2018 Feb 20;8(1):3335.

Toden S, Goel A, Restor J. The holy grail of curcumin and its efficacy in various diseases: is bioavailability truly a big concern? *Restor Med.* 2017 Dec;6(1):27-36.

Goel A. Utilizing biomarkers in colorectal cancer: an interview with Ajay Goel. *Future Oncol.* 2017 Dec;13(28):2511-2514.

Yoshida K, Toden S, Goel A et al. Curcumin sensitizes pancreatic cancer cells to gemcitabine by attenuating PRC2 subunit EZH2, and the lncRNA PVT1 expression. *Carcinogenesis.* 2017 Oct 1;38(10):1036-1046.

Toden S, Theiss AL, Goel A et al. Essential turmeric oils enhance anti-inflammatory efficacy of curcumin in dextran sulfate sodium-induced colitis. *Sci Rep.* 2017 Apr 11;7(1):814.

Shakibael M, Kraehe P, Goel A et al. Curcumin potentiates antitumor activity of 5-fluorouracil in a 3D alginate tumor microenvironment of colorectal cancer. *BMC Cancer.* 2015 Apr 10;15:250.

Toden SC, Goel A et al. Novel Evidence for Curcumin and Boswellic Acid-Induced Chemoprevention through Regulation of miR-34a and miR-27a in Colorectal Cancer. *Cancer Prev Res (Phila).* 2015 May;8(5):431-43.

Toden S, Okugawa Y, Goel A et al. Curcumin mediates chemosensitization to 5-fluorouracil through miRNA-induced suppression of epithelial-to-mesenchymal transition in chemoresistant colorectal cancer. *Carcinogenesis.* 2015 Mar;36(3):355-67.

Buhrmann C, Krehe P, Goel A et al. Curcumin suppresses crosstalk between colon cancer stem cells and stromal fibroblasts in the tumor microenvironment: potential role of EMT. *PLoS One.* 2014 Sep 19;9(9):e107514.

Shakibael M, Burhmann C, Goel A et al. Curcumin chemosensitizes 5-fluorouracil resistant MMR-deficient human colon cancer cells in high density cultures. *PLoS One.* 2014 Jan 3;9(1):e85397.

Sanmukhani J, Satodia V, Goel A et al. Efficacy and safety of curcumin in major depressive disorder: a randomized controlled trial. *Phytother Res.* 2014 Apr;28(4):579-85.

Link A, Balaguer F, Goel A et al. Curcumin modulates DNA methylation in colorectal cancer cells. *PLoS One.* 2013;8(2):e57709.

Shakibael M, Mobasheri A, Goel A et al. Curcumin enhances the effect of chemotherapy against colorectal cancer cells by inhibition of NF-κB and Src protein kinase signaling pathways. *PLoS One.* 2013;8(2):e57218.

Chandran B, Goel A. A randomized, pilot study to assess the efficacy and safety of curcumin in patients with active rheumatoid arthritis. *Phytother Res.* 2012 Nov;26(11):1719-25.

Reuter S, Gupta SC, Goel A et al. Epigenetic changes induced by curcumin and other natural compounds. *Genes Nutr.* 2011 May;6(2):93-108.

Goel A, Aggarwal BB. Curcumin, the golden spice from Indian saffron, is a chemosensitizer and radiosensitizer for tumors and chemoprotector and radioprotector for normal organs. *Nutr Cancer.* 2010;62(7):919-30.

Goel A, Jhurani S. Aggarwal BB. Multi-targeted therapy by curcumin: how spicy is it? *Mol Nutr Food Res.* 2008 Sep;52(9):1010-30.

Giros A, Grzybowski M, Goel A et al. Regulation of colorectal cancer cell apoptosis by the n-3 polyunsaturated fatty acids Docosahexaenoic and Eicosapentaenoic. *Cancer Prev Res (Phila).* 2009 Aug;2(8):732-42.

Goel A, Kunnumakkara AB, Aggarwal BB. Curcumin as "Curecumin": from kitchen to clinic. *Biochem Pharmacol.* 2008 Feb 15;75(4):787-809.

About the Authors

Dr. Ajay Goel

Dynamic and passionate—with a formidable record of patented innovations in cancer care—Ajay Goel, Ph.D., AGAF, is committed to developing better methods for the early detection and precision treatment of cancer. He joined City of Hope in June 2019 as founding chair of the new Department of Molecular Diagnostics and Experimental Therapeutics and founding director of Biotech Innovations at Beckman Research Institute.

A noted expert in gastrointestinal and other cancers, Dr. Goel is currently developing early-detection blood tests for colon, pancreatic and ovarian cancers—as well as a test for pancreatic cancer that can detect the disease seven years earlier than is now possible. Within the next few years, these tests are expected to become a simple and affordable part of everyone's annual health physical, just like tests for diabetes or cholesterol.

He is also working with genomic-based precision oncology to provide answers to the question: Why do therapies work with some good candidates and not with others?

Dr. Goel was born in India, received his Ph.D. in biophysics from Punjab University, completed his postgraduate work at the University of California, San Diego, and went on to a noteworthy 16-year career at Baylor Scott & White Research

Institute in Texas. He has authored more than 300 articles in peer-reviewed international journals and holds more than 30 advanced genomic and transcriptomic international patents.

Dr. Goel is a member of the American Association for Cancer Research and the American Gastroenterology Association and is on the international editorial boards of *World Journal of Gastroenterology* and *World Journal of Gastrointestinal Oncology.* He also performs peer-reviewing activities for almost 50 scientific journals, as well as serves on various grant-funding committees of the National Institutes of Health.

Terry Lemerond:

Terry Lemerond is a natural health expert with over 50 years of experience. He has owned health food stores, founded dietary supplement companies, and formulated over 400 products.

A much sought-after speaker and accomplished author, Terry shares his wealth of experience and knowledge in health and nutrition through social media, newsletters, podcasts, webinars, and personal speaking engagements. His books include *Seven Keys to Vibrant Health* and the sequel, *Seven Keys to Unlimited Personal Achievement,* and his newest publication, *50+ Natural Health Secrets Proven to Change Your Life.* His continual dedication, energy, and zeal are part of his on-going mission—to improve the health of America.

Index

KNOWLEDGE IS POWER,
ESPECIALLY FOR YOUR HEALTH!

re you in search of a reliable, science-based
esource for all your health and nutrition questions?
erry Talks Nutrition has you covered.

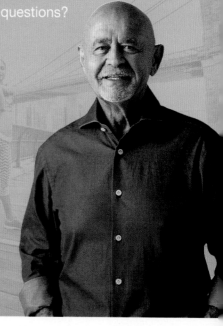

onnect with Terry to increase your
nowledge on a wide variety of topics,
cluding immunity, pain, curcumin and
ancer, diabetes, and so much more!

EAD
t
ryTalksNutrition.com
today's latest and
atest health and
rition information.

LISTEN
Tune in on Sat. and
Sun. 8-9 am (CST) at
TerryTalksNutrition.com for
a live internet radio show
hosted by Terry! You can
listen to past shows on the
website or on your favorite
podcast app.

ENGAGE
Connect with us on
Facebook, where you
can engage with other
individuals seeking safe
and effective ways to
improve overall wellness.

WATCH
Check out our
educational YouTube
Channel to learn from
the world's leading
doctors and health
experts.

Simply open your smartphone camera. Hold over desired code above for more information.

et answers to all of your health questions at **TERRYTALKSNUTRITION.COM**

WELCOME TO

ttn
publishing

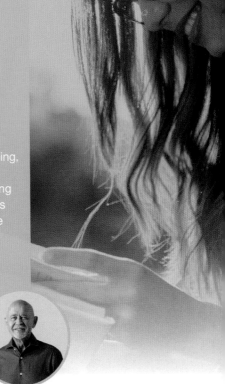

Are you ready to learn how anyone can use natural medicines, safely and effectively, to improve their health? You'll love TTN Publishing, my newest endeavor to bring you cutting edge research on powerful, health-supporting botanicals. I've coauthored numerous books with top alternative doctors from around the world to help you learn all you can about taking your health into your own hands. These educational books, supported by powerful scientific research, contain all the information you need to live a life of vibrant health.

In Good Health,
Terry Lemerond

BROUGHT TO YOU BY TTN PUBLISHING:

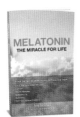
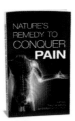
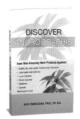
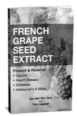

Get a copy for yourself and gift them to the people you care about!

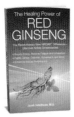
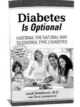
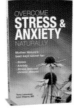
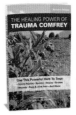
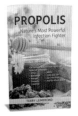

Available at your local health food store or online.

Visit TTNPublishing.com for more news and our latest publications.

TTNPUBLISHING.COM | info@ttnpublishing.com